DEADLY DISEASES AND EPIDEMICS

LEPROSY

Anthrax

Botulism

Campylobacteriosis

Cholera

Ebola

Encephalitis

Escherichia coli Infections

Gonorrhea

Hepatitis

Herpes

HIV/AIDS

Human Papillomavirus and Warts

Influenza

Leprosy

Lyme Disease

Mad Cow Disease (Bovine Spongiform Encephalopathy)

Malaria

Meningitis

Mononucleosis

Pelvic Inflammatory Disease

Plague

Polio

Salmonella

SARS

Smallpox

Streptococcus (Group A)

Staphylococcus aureus Infections

Syphilis

Toxic Shock Syndrome

Tuberculosis

Typhoid Fever

West Nile Virus

DEADLY DISEASES AND EPIDEMICS

LEPROSY

Alfica Sehgal

FOUNDING EDITOR
The Late **I. Edward Alcamo**
Distinguished Teaching Professor of Microbiology,
SUNY Farmingdale

FOREWORD BY
David Heymann
World Health Organization

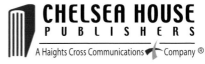

CHELSEA HOUSE
PUBLISHERS
A Haights Cross Communications Company ®
Philadelphia

CHELSEA HOUSE PUBLISHERS
VP, New Product Development Sally Cheney
Director of Production Kim Shinners
Creative Manager Takeshi Takahashi
Manufacturing Manager Diann Grasse

Staff for Leprosy
Executive Editor Tara Koellhoffer
Associate Editor Beth Reger
Editorial Assistant Kuorkor Dzani
Production Editor Bonnie Cohen
Photo Editor Sarah Bloom
Series Designer Terry Mallon
Cover Designer Keith Trego
Layout 21st Century Publishing and Communications, Inc.

http://www.chelseahouse.com

First Printing

1 3 5 7 9 8 6 4 2

Library of Congress Cataloging-in-Publication Data

Sehgal, Alfica.
  Leprosy/Alfica Sehgal.
    p. cm.—(Deadly diseases and epidemics)
  Includes bibliographical references and index.
  ISBN 0-7910-8502-3
  1. Leprosy. I. Title. II. Series.
  RC154.S38 2005
  614.5'46—dc22

                                        2005010391

Table of Contents

Foreword

In the 1960s, many of the infectious diseases that had terrorized generations were tamed. After a century of advances, the leading killers of Americans both young and old were being prevented with new vaccines or cured with new medicines. The risk of death from pneumonia, tuberculosis (TB), meningitis, influenza, whooping cough, and diphtheria declined dramatically. New vaccines lifted the fear that summer would bring polio, and a global campaign was on the verge of eradicating smallpox worldwide. New pesticides like DDT cleared mosquitoes from homes and fields, thus reducing the incidence of malaria, which was present in the southern United States and which remains a leading killer of children worldwide. New technologies produced safe drinking water and removed the risk of cholera and other water-borne diseases. Science seemed unstoppable. Disease seemed destined to all but disappear.

But the euphoria of the 1960s has evaporated.

The microbes fought back. Those causing diseases like TB and malaria evolved resistance to cheap and effective drugs. The mosquito developed the ability to defuse pesticides. New diseases emerged, including AIDS, Legionnaires, and Lyme disease. And diseases which had not been seen in decades re-emerged, as the hantavirus did in the Navajo Nation in 1993. Technology itself actually created new health risks. The global transportation network, for example, meant that diseases like West Nile virus could spread beyond isolated regions and quickly become global threats. Even modern public health protections sometimes failed, as they did in 1993 in Milwaukee, Wisconsin, resulting in 400,000 cases of the digestive system illness cryptosporidiosis. And, more recently, the threat from smallpox, a disease believed to be completely eradicated, has returned along with other potential bioterrorism weapons such as anthrax.

The lesson is that the fight against infectious diseases will never end.

In our constant struggle against disease, we as individuals have a weapon that does not require vaccines or drugs, and that is the warehouse of knowledge. We learn from the history of science that "modern" beliefs can be wrong. In this series of books, for example, you will learn that diseases like syphilis were once thought to be caused by eating potatoes. The invention of the microscope set science on the right path. There are more positive lessons from history. For example, smallpox was eliminated by vaccinating everyone who had come in contact with an infected person. This "ring" approach to smallpox control is still the preferred method for confronting an outbreak, should the disease be intentionally reintroduced.

At the same time, we are constantly adding new drugs, new vaccines, and new information to the warehouse. Recently, the entire human genome was decoded. So too was the genome of the parasite that causes malaria. Perhaps by looking at the microbe and the victim through the lens of genetics we will be able to discover new ways to fight malaria, which remains the leading killer of children in many countries.

Because of advances in our understanding of such diseases as AIDS, entire new classes of anti-retroviral drugs have been developed. But resistance to all these drugs has already been detected, so we know that AIDS drug development must continue.

Education, experimentation, and the discoveries that grow out of them are the best tools to protect health. Opening this book may put you on the path of discovery. I hope so, because new vaccines, new antibiotics, new technologies, and, most importantly, new scientists are needed now more than ever if we are to remain on the winning side of this struggle against microbes.

David Heymann
Executive Director
Communicable Diseases Section
World Health Organization
Geneva, Switzerland

1

Historical Overview

"My life could have been so different and maybe a lot shorter" said Hari, a young man from a rural village in India. He was found to have contracted *kushtha* when he was only nine years old. As was often the case with this disease, he was about to be abandoned by his family, until a very open-minded doctor found out about him. Luckily, the boy did not have a severely infective form of the disease and his family was not at risk. Still, everyone in his village was too frightened to touch him. They called him cursed and wanted nothing to do with him. They only knew that something terrible was making people in their village very ill. Fortunately, the doctor succeeded in allaying the villagers' fears, and, after many sessions and conversations with almost half of the villagers, the boy was able to remain with his family. He was properly treated, and soon, the only reminder of the disease we know as leprosy was a tiny scar on his back. Listening to this young man of 20, today, it is obvious that, in addition to its physical symptoms, the disease also brought the devastating pain of social stigma. The fear of being left alone also had a positive effect, however. It helped him to become a social worker, which is a matter of pride for him today. He has been teaching biology in a school for several years, and his own life experience has certainly helped him reach out to his students.

Kushtha, the name by which leprosy, or Hansen's disease, is known in India, is also the name used to document the disease in very early scriptures of ancient Indian civilization. No matter what it is called, leprosy is caused by a bacterium called *Mycobacterium leprae*, a microscopic germ, which is closely related to the tuberculosis bacillus. Like tuberculosis, it is transmitted through breathing—through droplets emitted by a person with an active case of the disease. Unlike tuberculosis, however, it is not highly contagious. Most people (90–95%) have a genetic immunity to leprosy, and leprosy experts generally say that prolonged and intimate contact with a contagious individual is required for a susceptible person to acquire the disease.

The disease principally affects nerves and skin, with other organs of the body being affected only in late stages. Germs may be spread through coughing and sneezing. Many patients develop deformities due to nerve damage, as the disease runs its course. Contrary to popular misconceptions, leprosy does not cause limbs to fall off or flesh to rot. The bacillus does, however, damage the peripheral nerves, causing insensitivity or lack of feeling. Nerve damage is the major cause of disability associated with leprosy. The painlessness that results from nerve damage allows affected individuals to ignore cuts, burns, and other injuries sustained during everyday activities. These injuries may become infected or even **gangrenous,** and amputation is required in some cases. As a result of these deformities, patients are often isolated, affecting their social and economic well-being. According to a statistics in 1991 an estimated 6 million people worldwide are infected with leprosy.

Until the discovery of **AIDS** (acquired immune deficiency syndrome), leprosy was the most feared infectious disease in the world. Even today, however, leprosy's effects still drastically change the lives of millions of people—living mainly in Asia, South America, and Africa. Brazil is the second-most affected nation, after India.

In the last half of the 14th century, leprosy swept though Europe, killing one-third of the population, but it came and went quickly, like a great earthquake, followed by a series of aftershocks. Today, the disease is most prevalent in underprivileged areas, where crowded and unsanitary conditions contribute to its spread. Leprosy has even been known to develop in more developed nations, from time to time. In the United States, the disease is found mainly in Louisiana, Texas, Florida, Hawaii, and California. It can also be found in the Northeast, however, and other areas where immigrants from **endemic** areas have settled.

LEPROSY: THE HIDDEN DISEASE

When the rash on his chest first appeared, the 48-year-old office worker dismissed it as an allergic reaction to the shellfish he had recently eaten. His doctor agreed and prescribed an ointment. But when the red bumps did not go away after several months and began to spread to his legs, arms, and face, the man began to worry. He saw another doctor, who had no explanation for his condition, and finally another, who gave him a startling diagnosis: leprosy.

In the United States, leprosy is usually regarded as a plague of the past, a disease relegated to biblical times or, perhaps, to poor and distant countries. In fact, as cases of leprosy have been declining worldwide in recent years, the infection has actually been on the rise in the United States. While there were some 900 recorded cases in the United States 40 years ago, today more than 7,000 people have leprosy, or Hansen's disease, as it is now called.

The disease, even with its sanitized name, can still confer pariah status on the victim. Thus, there is no sign on the door announcing a clinic in New York, even though it has almost 500 people receiving regular outpatient care and is one of only 11 federal Hansen's disease centers. On a recent morning, a sampling of patients, all of them wishing to remain anonymous, said they were loath to tell others about their diagnoses.

A Queens, New York, man tells his friends that the bumpy patches on his arms are allergies, and a stylish college student has kept her infection secret from everyone but her grandmother. A 61-year-old Staten Island

Although, there is an effective treatment for the disease, the number of cases in the United States is still significant. The World Health Organization (WHO) is working to eradicate the disease worldwide.

man who is being treated for a recurrence of leprosy he first contracted 40 years ago says he still has not told his wife of 33 years.

Most of those infected in the United States are immigrants from global leprosy hot spots—Brazil, India, and the Caribbean, for example. In the past six years, however, a few patients at the New York clinic—including a 73-year-old man from Queens, who had never been out of the country, and an elderly Jewish man from Westchester County—have contracted leprosy in the United States.

As a result, the disease is now officially endemic to the Northeastern United States for the first time ever. (Cases of leprosy transmission in the Southeast date as far back as the turn of the 19th century.) Leprosy experts think that even some foreign-born people with the infection may have acquired it in immigrant communities here.

Leprosy's symptoms—bumpy rashes, skin indentations, and loss of feeling in hands and feet—are often misdiagnosed as being caused by a variety of disorders, including bug bites and lupus. Promptly recognized, the disease is relatively easy to treat. With a standard regimen of multiple drugs, a vast majority of people with leprosy cease to be contagious within three months and become free of the bacteria that cause it in two to five years. Without treatment, however, the disease can be spread. The bacteria are thought to be passed through the respiratory droplets of an infected person. Untreated infections can also result in serious complications, including the loss of toes or limbs.

Leprosy is also known as Hansen's disease, after Gerhard Armauer Hansen, the Norwegian scientist who first observed the bacillus under a microscope in 1873, and identified it as the cause of leprosy. The disease shares a unique history with human beings, because, unlike most communicable diseases, *Mycobacterium leprae* has virtually only one host— the human body.

HISTORY OF THE DISEASE

Leprosy has affected humans since the dawn of history, leaving lasting imprints on religion, literature, and the arts. It is a deep-rooted part of the human psyche, with both mystical and physical meanings. Asians and Africans call it "the big disease," because of the damage it does to the soul and body of the patient (Figure 1.1).

Leprosy appears in the Old Testament of the Bible (as the Hebrew word *tzaraath*) and it probably covered a whole range of horrible skin conditions, just as the Greek word *lepra* did in the New Testament, where the words *leprous* or *leprosy* appear 54 times. These biblical accounts resulted in the disease being linked to corruption of both the spirit and the body. The book of Leviticus paints a chilling image of this disease: "And the leper in whom the plague is, his clothes shall be rent, and the hair of his head shall go loose, and he shall cover his upper lip, and shall cry, unclean, unclean. And all the days wherein the plague is in him he shall be unclean; he is unclean: he shall dwell alone; without the camp shall his dwelling be."[1]

The Bible equated leprosy with sin. The disease was seen as a punishment from God, for some transgression. According to the Old Testament, Uzziah, the king of Judah, wanted to burn incense in the temple of Jehovah, a ceremony reserved for priests. The priests opposed him, and, the story goes, Uzziah became angry, so God struck him with leprosy. King Uzziah, was a leper until the day of his death, and dwelt in a separate house. He was cut off from the house of Jehovah. The priests did not drive Uzziah into the wilderness, like lesser sinners. Instead, they stripped him of power and denied him burial in the cemetery of kings. The New Testament treats lepers

ARMAUER HANSEN AND THE DISCOVERY OF LEPROSY

A prominent dermatologist in Norway, Daniel Cornelius Danielsen, wrote the first extensive description of leprosy in 1847; it was this description that Norwegian physician Armauer Hansen used 20 years later as the basis for his studies of leprosy. Up to this time, researchers had been unable to infect laboratory animals with the disease, nor were they able to grow the bacteria in culture. Still unsure what caused leprosy, Hansen undertook a bold approach to uncovering what caused the disease: He took tissue samples from people infected with leprosy and implanted this tissue into healthy nurses, patients, and other individuals. Hansen's experiments did not result in any healthy individuals becoming sick, but they did result in harsh legal condemnation for the maverick research physician.

Nevertheless, Hansen remained committed to discovering the cause of the dreaded disease and, in 1873, succeeded in isolating and identifying *Mycobacterium leprae* under the microscope (eight years before Koch successfully isolated and identified the bacterium that causes human tuberculosis). Hansen garnered the recognition he so deserved in 1909, when he was honored at the Second International Leprosy Congress in Bergen, Norway. Today, Hansen's name endures through the Armauer Hansen Research Institute in Ethiopia, which is committed to eradicating and treating leprosy and also to educating leprosy field specialists.

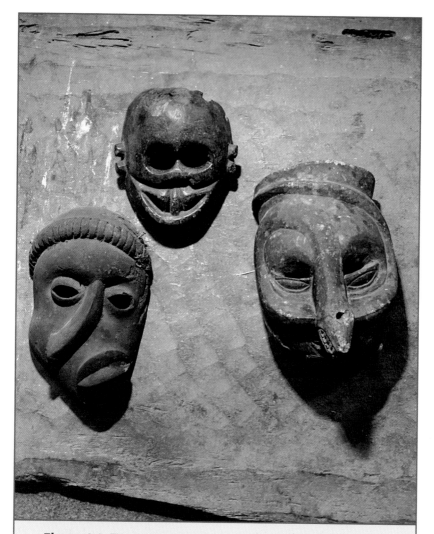

Figure 1.1 These ancient masks show the deformities that many ancient cultures had associated with leprosy. Having leprosy caused a person to be isolated and shunned from the community.

more kindly, but still sets them apart from other sufferers. Jesus healed the blind and deaf, but cleansed the lepers, implying that there was some moral stigma associated with the disease. In biblical literature, segregation and disinfection were mentioned as methods to contain the disease. The one thing that we know for sure about leprosy is that it is a very old disease, spanning back to biblical times.

One account of a disease that could be leprosy appears in an Egyptian papyrus inscribed about 1552–1350 B.C.E., but no one really knows for sure whether the disease being described was actually leprosy. Examination of mummies in Egypt indicates that the disease existed in that country as early as the 2nd century B.C.E. It is believed that, in the

SPECIAL MASS

There was a special mass performed in the Middle Ages in Western Europe, at the site of a newly identified leper's hut. Sometimes referred to as a Mass of Separation, one such version of the mass as spoken by the priest is as follows:

I forbid you to enter the church or monastery, fair, mill, market-place, or company of persons...ever to leave your house without your leper's costume [a white robe to cover the body] and a bell in hand...to wash your hands or anything about you in the stream or fountain. I forbid you to enter a tavern...I forbid you, if you go on the road and you meet some person who speaks to you, to fail to put yourself downwind before you answer...I forbid you to go into a narrow lane so that if you should meet anyone he might catch the affliction from you...I forbid you ever to touch children or give them anything. I forbid you to eat or drink from any dishes but your own. I forbid you to eat or drink in company, unless with lepers.*

Ignorance about the disease led people to associate it with sins and dirt. Thus, separation of the patients from the rest of society seemed the only logical choice.

* *Acta Leprol.*, 2001 12:79–84.

1st century B.C.E., following fighting in Egypt, Roman soldiers of the army of Pompey, carried the disease with them when they traveled from Egypt to Italy. It is also thought that, in the Middle Ages, the disease spread from Italy, throughout the rest of Europe.

The disease took on epidemic proportions in the 13th century, during the Crusades. Advancing troops and pilgrims are believed to have spread the disease, even to Jerusalem, where King Baudouin is reported to have suffered from leprosy. The disease has never been geographically localized to any one particular area of the world, as evidenced by the fact that it probably existed in India and in Japan before 1000 B.C.E.

Leprosy is mentioned (as kushtha) by the renowned Indian physician, Sushruta, in his book *Sushruta Samhita* as early as 600 B.C.E. There is some doubt, however, whether kushtha meant leprosy, as we know it today. The disease also appears in the records of ancient Greece, when the army of Alexander the Great returned from India, in 326 B.C.E. In Rome, the first mention coincides with the return of Pompey's troops from Asia Minor in 62 B.C.E. Asia, therefore, could have been the cradle of infection, before it spread throughout most of Europe.

During the Middle Ages in Europe, patients were segregated into thousands of centers, which came to be known as lazarets or leprosarias. As mentioned earlier, containment was naturally considered the most practical means of controlling the disease. Leprosy came to be referred to as "the living death" and its victims were actually treated as though they had already died. Funeral services were conducted to declare their "death" to society. Psychologically, victims of untreated leprosy could actually develop a self-loathing, where they imagined that, at heart, they were unclean and under some sort of curse. Other cruel practices required the leprosy patient to walk on a particular side of the road, depending which way the wind was blowing. In some areas in Europe, people with the disease were required by law to dress in special clothing, wear a declaration sign around their neck, and ring a warning bell announcing that they were "lepers," and people should flee. Other equally discriminating laws of church and state required the use of separate seats in churches, separate holy water vessels, and, in some cases in Britain, there was a "lepers' slot" in the church wall through which the "leper" could view the communion service, but not "contaminate" the service by his presence.

Around the end of the 15th century, leprosy ceased to be endemic, with the exception of Norway and the Mediterranean. It seems certain, however, that Spanish conquerors in the slave trade, together with French-speaking colonialists who were forced out of Nova Scotia in the middle of the 18th century, to settle in the southern United States, helped to spread *M. leprae* to the American continent. From Europe, in the early part of the 20th century, the European colonialists seem to have taken the disease to certain islands in the Pacific Ocean, particularly Nauru, in the southwestern Pacific Ocean, about 2,580 miles (4,160 km) southwest of Hawaii.[2]

ATTEMPTS TOWARD DEVELOPING REMEDIES

In ancient times, containment was thought the only way to eventually find a cure, but as human minds developed over time, people started to think of other curative measures, as well. Finding a cure became even more important when the infected person was of significant stature in the community. In Burma, according to legend, when the king of Burma contracted leprosy, he was advised by the gods to eat the fruit from the Kalaw tree, which was said to have cured him. In reality, chaulmoogra oil extracted from the nut of this particular tree had been used as a treatment for centuries, with little real success.

For centuries, leprosy continued to take its toll in India, and many patients were banished and sometimes killed. In

Hindu mythology, the god Rama is said to have contracted kushtha, but was cured by taking a medicine made from the fruit of the chaulmoogra tree. The same fruit was rumored to have been effective in China.

In 1853, Dr. J.F. Mouat, of the Bengal Medical Service was presented with a drunken, filthy beggar, who obviously had kushtha. Mouat remembered the famous Hindu epic about the god Rama being cured by the fruit of the chaulmoogra tree and had an interest in Indian herbal medicines, so he decided to administer the crushed chaulmoogra seeds six times a day to the sick man. He was so impressed by the improvement in the beggar's health, that he wrote an article of his trials for the *Indian Medical Journal*. He also shared some of the oil with medical colleagues serving in Mauritius. News of the value of this oil, sometimes also called hydno-carpus oil, spread throughout the world, and experiments were also carried out in Egypt to test its effectiveness against the *M. leprae* bacterium.

Around the same time, an Irish adventurer named Wellesley Bailey, traveled to Australia and New Zealand, in a futile search for gold and a fortune in farming. He eventually found his way to India, where he planned to join the police force in Faizabad, in what is now Uttar Pradesh, in the northern part of India. The police force, however, did not hold his interest for long and he drifted into missionary service. The American Presbyterian Mission appointed him as a teacher in one of its schools in northwest India. He was later appointed as a volunteer to take care of lepers. He wrote, "If there was ever a Christ-like work in the world, it is to go amongst these poor sufferers and bring them the consolation of the Gospel."[3]

Wellesley Bailey's girlfriend, Alice Grahame, lived in Dublin and shared with her friends—the three Pim sisters, Isabella, Charlotte, and Jan—some of her letters from Wellesley. The letters told of the terrible suffering of those with leprosy.

Wellesley and Alice were married in Bombay and continued their missionary work for many years. The Baileys eventually resigned from missionary service and returned to Ireland where, in 1874, something occurred that would have wonderful repercussions for leprosy patients in India.

The three Pim sisters were so shocked and moved by the stories recounted in Wellesley's letters, that they resolved to produce an informational booklet containing 16 chapters, entitled *Lepers in India*. This meager first step led to the formation of The Mission to Lepers, later to be named The Leprosy Mission, a pioneer organization for modern leprosy work in India.

One year earlier, in 1873, Dr. Armauer Hansen, a Norwegian scientist had discovered the cause of leprosy. At the time, many thought leprosy was a "curse of God," but Hansen demonstrated that a bacterium—*Mycobacterium leprae*—which was spreading in a frightening manner in Norway, was the real culprit (Figure 1.2). In 1875, the Baileys returned to India. This time, Wellesley Bailey was a lay-missionary, employed by the Church of Scotland. Sadly, the mission refused to accept the Baileys' ministry to lepers as part of the Gospel. The Baileys left the Church of Scotland Mission to more fully establish The Mission to Lepers. Today, this same mission, renamed Leprosy Mission International, is one of the largest agencies treating leprosy patients in 30 countries—with over 100 hospitals-clinics in India alone.

With the 1898 Leper Act, issued by the British government in India, "lepers" were treated like animals, condemned to suffer compulsory segregation in asylums or "leper colonies." The Mission to Lepers offered loving, compassionate care at Purulia, West Bengal, where, later, the mission's headquarters for all of India and Southern Asia was established. By the end of the 17th century, over 600 lepers were accommodated at Purulia, where the mission provided free education, comfortable living quarters, and limited medical

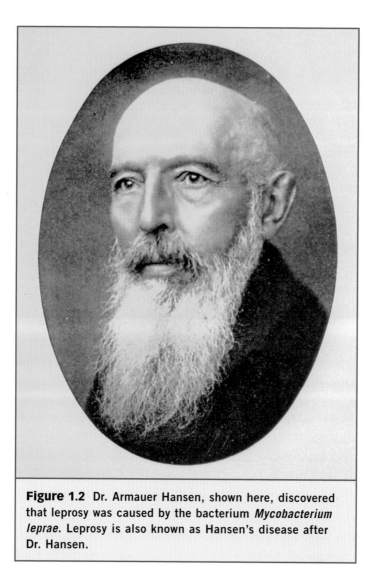

Figure 1.2 Dr. Armauer Hansen, shown here, discovered that leprosy was caused by the bacterium *Mycobacterium leprae*. Leprosy is also known as Hansen's disease after Dr. Hansen.

and surgical treatment. (At the time, chaulmoogra oil was the only drug available.)

Fortunately, the situation improved, somewhat. With developing scientific knowledge and technological abilities, things began to change for the better. Just how and when things changed will be described in greater detail in Chapter 6.

2

The Spread, Signs, and Types of Leprosy

As we learned in Chapter 1, leprosy can have devastating physical and psychological effects. Since biblical times, it has been one of the most feared and socially stigmatizing diseases in the world. To contract the disease, one has to live in close contact with an infected individual for a prolonged period. That said, in 2002, 763,917 new cases of leprosy were detected worldwide. It is, therefore, extremely important to recognize the early symptoms of leprosy, report them to medical authorities, start medication, and continue with treatment, once diagnosed. Many people all over the world remain undiagnosed or do not complete treatment, once they are diagnosed. Here is an example to elaborate on this problem:

In September 1999, Standwa Jama was diagnosed with leprosy. At the time, he was 12 years old. Standwa lived in the Eastern Cape Province of South Africa. The Leprosy Mission had been running a leprosy control program in the Eastern Cape, since 1981. Previously, there had been two leprosy hospitals in the province, but they were closed, as treatment began to focus more on home-based care and drug therapy (See Chapter 6). Standwa was found by The Leprosy Mission's program manager, Frikkie Naudé. According to Naudé's diagnosis, Standwa was suffering from multi-bacillary leprosy. Standwa came from a very poor family and was under the care of his aunt at the time of his diagnosis. He had never been to school and was herding the family's cattle. At first, Standwa was very frightened of Naudé and his medical team, but Naudé eventually managed to win his trust, and they developed a friendly relationship.

Unfortunately, Standwa's father came and took him away to the city about 1,000 kilometers (621 miles) away. Apparently, the father had found a small job for his son—and in a poor family, any income was a blessing. In the meantime, Standwa's illness would not be treated. Naudé and his team eventually found four other members of the family, who were also suffering from leprosy. Altogether, five members of the family were infected. Standwa's brother, Xolani, had leprosy, as did three of his cousins and his grandmother. Xolani was diagnosed in May 2001. At that time, Standwa reappeared at home and was able to resume treatment. At the time of his diagnosis, Xolani was being taunted by other children because of his swollen lips and nose. Swollen and flabby lips and facial parts are among the definitive signs of the disease. Being embarrassed by his disfigured face, Xolani had become socially aloof. He used to avoid mixing and playing with other children or interacting with anyone around till the treatment helped in his recovery. All five of the family members are now receiving treatment and returning to their normal live.

HOW IS THE DISEASE TRANSMITTED?

Throughout history, leprosy has been regarded as contagious and those affected have been secluded and barred from society. People feared that merely touching an infected person could spread the disease. Today, scientists know that leprosy is not so easily transmitted, but the exact mechanism of transmission of *M. leprae* is still a mystery.

There are, however, theories about the possible ways the disease is spread, including direct person-to-person contact, or contact with respiratory secretions from infected individuals. When an infected but untreated person sneezes, their nasal secretions may contain large numbers of leprosy bacteria. Conceivably, these released bacteria can be inhaled by a healthy individual or could invade a healthy person's body through a cut or abrasion on the skin, infecting that person. There is some evidence that contact with infected soil may also be a method of transmission. It is important to note that most people will never develop the disease, even if they are exposed to the bacteria. In fact, 95% of the world population is immune to the bacteria that cause leprosy. Although the exact reasons for these differences are not completely understood, bad nutrition, unhygienic habits, constitutional conditions (tuberculosis, alcoholism) seem to favor its production and propagation.

Unlike other contagious diseases, such as influenza and cholera, patients who receive treatment for leprosy do not generally spread the disease, once treated. When a person with leprosy is placed on medication, most of the bacteria in their body dies off within a few days. Within a couple of weeks after starting the medicine, the risk of transferring the disease is negligible. Today, doctors believe that it is not necessary to isolate a person with leprosy after the medical treatment has begun. It is also important to note that the disease is not transmitted sexually or from a pregnant mother to her fetus. Very rarely do healthcare workers who care for patients with leprosy develop the disease. The well-known case of Father Damien, a Belgian missionary who contracted the disease while caring for leprosy patients on the Hawaiian island of Molokai, during the late 1800s, appears to be the exception, rather than the rule (Figure 2.1).

SIGNS AND SYMPTOMS OF LEPROSY

Like most other diseases, early recognition or detection of leprosy is very important. Early treatment can limit damage caused by the disease, render the person noninfectious, and allow the patient to lead a normal life. The most common first sign is usually a spot on the skin that may be slightly red, darker, or **hypopigmented** (lighter in color than the rest of the skin). The spot often develops **anaesthesia** (loss of sensation) and may lose hair. Some of these spots may slowly increase in size and new spots may appear on other parts of the body. Most

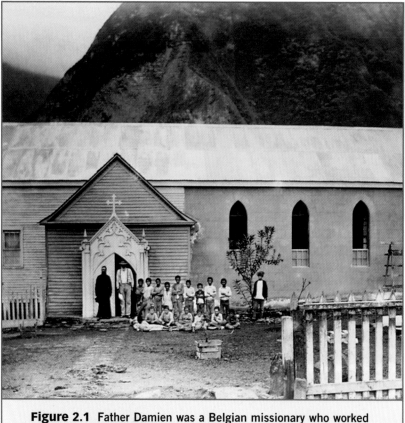

Figure 2.1 Father Damien was a Belgian missionary who worked with leprosy patients on the Hawaiian island of Molokai. He is seen here standing in front of his church with the patients that he treated. Father Damien contracted leprosy and eventually died of the disease.

often, spots appear on the arms, legs, or back. Skin lesions that do not heal within several weeks of an injury are a typical sign of leprosy. The order in which symptoms appear in a particular body part is not completely understood.

As the disease progresses, patients can develop enlarged peripheral nerves, usually near joints, such as the wrist, elbow, and knees. Next, nerves in different body parts start to be affected. If the arms are the infected limbs, part of the hand can become numb and small muscles can become paralyzed, lead-ing to the curling of the fingers and thumb (Figure 2.2). When the disease attacks the nervous system in the legs, it interrupts sensation in the feet. If facial nerves are affected, a person loses the blinking reflex of the eyes, which can eventually lead to dryness, ulceration, and blindness. Bacilli entering the mucous lining of the nose can lead to internal damage and scarring

FATHER DAMIEN

Father Damien lived from 1840 to 1889, and was originally named Joseph Damien de Veuster. He was one of Hawaii's most illustrious citizens. A Belgian missionary priest, he went to Hawaii in 1864, as a Picpus Father (priest of the Sacred Heart of Jesus and Mary). He was ordained in Honolulu and worked among the islanders for several years. In 1873, at his request, he was sent to the lepers' colony of Kalaupapa on the island of Molokai. There, he labored until his death from leprosy. A dedicated and driven man, Father Damien did more than simply administer the faith. He built homes, churches, and coffins; arranged for medical services and funding from Honolulu, and became a parent to children whose own parents had died. A statue of Father Damien, created by artist Marisol Escobar, stands in Statuary Hall in Washington, D.C.

Kalaupapa's reputation as a leper colony is well known. Leprosy is believed to have spread to Hawaii from China. The first documented case of leprosy occurred in 1848. Its rapid spread and unknown cure precipitated the urgent need for complete and total isolation of its victims. Surrounded on three sides by the Pacific Ocean and cut off from the rest of Molokai by 1,600-foot (488-m) sea cliffs, Kalaupapa provided the perfect isolated environment. In early 1866, the first leprosy victims were shipped to Kalaupapa and lived there for seven years before Father Damien arrived.

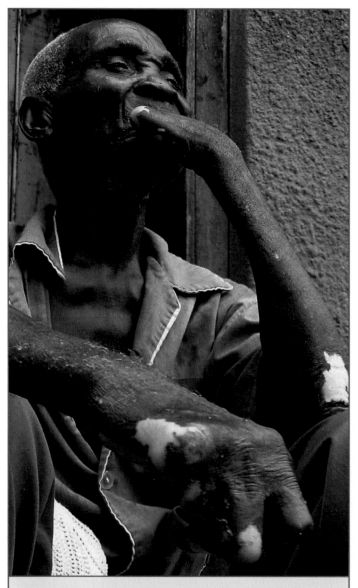

Figure 2.2 The man in this picture is afflicted with leprosy, which has damaged his hands and arms. Leprosy causes white patches of skin and numbing of the nerves in the body, which can lead to damage of the extremities such as the fingers and toes.

that, in time, causes the nose to collapse. The muscles get weaker, resulting in signs such as foot drop (the toe drags when the foot is lifted to take a step). Muscle weakness, scars or lesions on body, loss of sensation from any discolored spot on the skin, and prolonged healing time for wounds are also indications that someone may be infected with leprosy bacteria. What makes the bacteria harm one body part over another is not clearly understood. Infection appears to be the result of interplay between the bacteria and the body's immune system.

DEFORMITIES AND LEPROSY

If the early signs go unnoticed and, thus, are not medicated, leprosy symptoms will start to intensify. Left untreated, leprosy can cause deformity, crippling, and blindness. Because the bacteria attack nerve endings, the terminal body parts (hands and feet) lose all sensations and cannot feel heat, touch, or pain, and can be easily injured. Patients end up hurting themselves—often severely—with fire, thorns, rocks, and even hot coffee cups. Left unattended, these wounds can then get further infected and cause tissue damage. Along with these injuries, fingers and toes become shortened and deformed, as the cartilage is absorbed into the body. Contrary to popular belief, the disease does not cause body parts to "fall off." In many patients, a large proportion of ulcers originate under callused or scarred skin. This callus, if not regularly removed, builds up and forms a thick mass, some of which dehydrates and becomes hard. On the sole of the foot, this may cause excessive pressure in the deeper tissues while walking, resulting in ulceration (Figure 2.3).

TYPES OF LEPROSY

Depending on the number of lesions and the number of bacillus observed on a lesion smear, leprosy can be classified into two groups: tuberculoid and lepromatous (also discussed in Chapter 5).

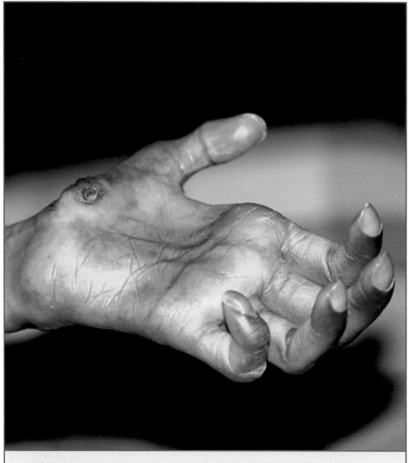

Figure 2.3 Leprosy can cause curling of the fingers as the muscles become paralyzed. It can also cause lesions to form, such as the one on the palm of this person's hand.

Tuberculoid Leprosy (TT)

In this form of the disease, the skin lesions appear as light red or purplish spots. Patients usually have one or a few (normally fewer than five) hypopigmented lesions with well-defined borders. **Tuberculoid leprosy** is the more benign type, even though the nerves are affected, which leads to numbness (usually of the extremities). This form affects the peripheral nerves and, sometimes, the surrounding skin, on the face, arms, legs, and buttocks. Sensory loss is frequently observed around the lesions. Tuberculoid leprosy is also known as **paucibacillary leprosy**. In this type, the nerve architecture is destroyed and there can be formation of **granulomas** in nerves. Granulomas (inflamed nodules caused by the infection) are visible at the clinical level, as asymmetric nerve enlargement near the skin lesion.

Lepromatous Leprosy

In this type, the skin lesions appear as yellow or brown nodules (protuberances), which are penetrated by many blood vessels. Usually, there are multiple, poorly defined, hypopigmented areas that affect the mucous membranes of the eyes, nose, and throat. Multiple **papules** (nodular elevations on the skin) can appear. These are usually symmetrically distributed and tend to infiltrate (penetrate) the skin. There is a general thickening of the skin, especially on the face and ears. Patients with an advanced form of this disease may lose eyelashes or eyebrows. When someone suffers from disfiguring facial features, this condition is known as **leonine facies**. **Lepromatous leprosy**, also called **multibacillary leprosy**, is the more easily spread of the two forms of leprosy. This more severe form produces large disfiguring nodules. The peripheral **neuropathy** (diseased state of the nerves) observed in lepromatous leprosy, causes muscle weakness and atrophy and has been associated with claw hands and foot drops. In this form, the nerve structure is not destroyed much, but the nodules present in the neural areas have numerous bacteria.

According to some classifications, there is another form of the disease, called **borderline leprosy**. This form is characterized by the presence of single or multiple skin lesions with ill-defined or indistinct borders. Many satellite lesions emerge around the larger ones. As suggested by the name, the nerve structure shows an intermediate kind of pathology, with some

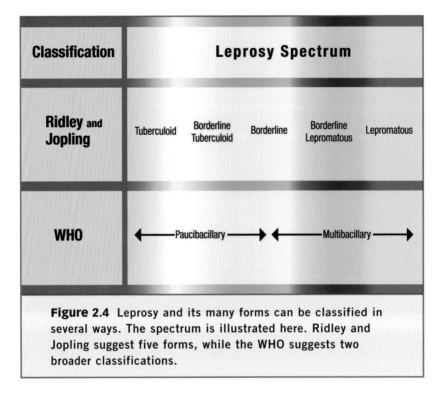

Figure 2.4 Leprosy and its many forms can be classified in several ways. The spectrum is illustrated here. Ridley and Jopling suggest five forms, while the WHO suggests two broader classifications.

damage, but not as much as is seen in the tuberculoid form. This form can, however, cause maximum nerve damage, as multiple nerves are involved. The nerve involvement is earlier and faster than in the lepromatous form.

Different people have found more and more elaborate ways to classify the disease and there are many intermediate forms described between the tubercuolid and lepromatous types. These forms are outlined in Figure 2.4.

3

Leprosy Around the World

Leprosy is the oldest recorded disease in history, and it continues to be a health challenge today. Prevalence of the disease has greatly decreased, through the use of multi-drug therapy approved by the World Health Organization (WHO) and vaccinations with BCG (Bacillus Calmette Guérin) (discussed in Chapter 4). Though rare in the United States, the disease is still a problem in parts of Texas and Louisiana, possibly due to the presence of the nine-banded armadillo. Although the only known reservoir for the bacteria that causes leprosy is humans, diseases caused by bacilli indistinguishable from *M. leprae* have been discovered in armadillos of the southern United States. There are approximately 7,000 people currently diagnosed with leprosy in the United States, and about 150 to 200 new cases are reported each year.[4] The American Leprosy Missions (ALM) helps to fund the U.S. Public Health Services' National Hansen's Disease Program, located in Baton Rouge, Louisiana.

At the beginning of 2004, the number of leprosy patients under treatment in the world was around 460,000. About 515,000 new cases were detected during 2003. Among them, 43% were multibacillary cases, 12% were in children, and 3% were diagnosed with severe disabilities. During the previous two years, the global number of new cases detected had continued to decrease dramatically (a reduction of about 20% per year).[5]

Information campaigns about leprosy in high-risk areas are crucial. Patients and their families, who have historically been ostracized from their communities, must be encouraged to come forward and receive treatment (Figure 3.1).

The problem of accurate diagnosis is further complicated by the inability to reach potentially infected areas. According to the WHO, there

Figure 3.1 Global Leprosy Situation in 2004*

WHO Region	Point Prevalence	Cases detected during year 2003
Africa	51,233	47,006
Americas	86,652	52,435
East Mediterranean	5,798	3,940
South East Asia	304,296	405,147
Western Pacific	10,449	6,190
WORLD	458,428	514,718

Figure 3.1 As of 2004, leprosy was most prevalent in South East Asia according to the World Health Organization (WHO). Throughout the world, there were over 400,000 cases of leprosy reported in 2004 alone. Most cases of leprosy are treatable, but people must be informed about the disease and where to seek treatment.

* Adapted from www.who.int/en/

are approximately 3,000 cases of leprosy in the African nation of Angola.[6] The actual number of cases, however, is most likely much higher. Inaccessible regions and land mines make accurate reporting difficult in many areas of Angola. Poverty and lack of education also contribute to the difficulty of properly diagnosing affected patients. Angola has one doctor for every 16,152 people. (The United States, in contrast, has one doctor for every 400 people)[7].

A similar example of inaccessibility to patients is seen in the Philippines. According to the WHO, approximately 4,250 cases of leprosy have been registered in the Philippines.[8] Its island geography, areas of high mountains, and deep jungles make accurate recording difficult in remote regions. Remarkably, around 80,000 people have been cured with drug therapy in the Philippines.[9] Although there are many countries with a relatively small incidence of the disease, the greater part of the global burden is now focused on the top six endemic countries: India, Brazil, Madagascar, Mozambique, Nepal, and Tanzania. The total number of cases registered in these six countries combined represents 83% of the global prevalence of the disease. The prevalence rate is 3.4 cases per 10,000 people. India alone represents around 64% of prevalence and 76% of new cases in the world.[10]

We have certainly come a very long way from the first International Leprosy Congress held in Berlin, Germany, in 1897. The only points on which all experts agreed at that time were that leprosy was incurable, and that the only immediate solution was to isolate patients. The first formal attempt to estimate the global leprosy epidemic was made by the WHO in 1966, resulting in an estimated total number of about 11 million cases, of which 60% of patients were not registered for treatment.[11] By the mid-1970s, it was obvious that efforts to control leprosy with long-term Dapsone drug therapy were failing. This realization led to the establishment of WHO/TDR research programs directed at development of an effective protective vaccine (known as IMMLEP) and more effective leprosy therapy (known as THELEP).

LEPROSY IS DIFFERENT

Compared to many other infectious diseases, leprosy is very different. This disease causes more pain and social trauma than even death itself. When we look at the leading causes of death worldwide: acute lower respiratory infection, tuberculosis, diarrhea (including dysentery), HIV/AIDS, malaria, measles, hepatitis B, pertussis (whooping cough), neonatal tetanus, and

MODERN TECHNIQUES DETECT LEPROSY IN ANCIENT SAMPLES

The human mind is always curious to know "when," "where," and "how" things happen. In an attempt to understand the spread of different diseases in ancient times, scientists have devised many methods of study, at the molecular level. The technique utilizes the unique features of the DNA of different organisms. The molecular biology method used predominantly for such experiments is called polymerase chain reaction (PCR). People have been trying to analyze archaeological material for the presence of pathogenic microorganisms like *Plasmodium* (responsible for malaria), *Schistosoma* (a worm causing schistosomasis), *M. tuberculosis* (causes tuberculosis), and *M. leprae* (the leprosy bacteria). Results from some of these experiments have demonstrated the presence of *M. tuberculosis* DNA in specimens from the 18th century, and even earlier. Some of this work was done using naturally mummified human remains from the 18th century in Vác, Hungary. Analyses done with samples from Dakhleh Oasis, Egypt (Roman period); 1st century Palestine; Poland and Hungary, dating from the 10th–11th centuries; and medieval Sweden show the presence of *M. leprae* DNA in specimens.

dengue (hemorrhagic fever), we see that leprosy does not even make the top ten. The issue with leprosy is not **mortality** rates, but, rather, its social stigma. We need to look at leprosy differently than we look at most other infectious diseases, focusing more on instilling in the public an awareness of the socially demoralizing aspect of the disease and its effects. With leprosy, compassion and educated social values would do just as much, if not more, than science and technology alone.

4

What Causes Leprosy?

Bacteria are single-celled organisms without a defined **nucleus** that exist all around us. They come in different shapes and sizes, occurring as singles or in groups. Some bacteria form chains, while others are in groups. These little creatures are an integrated part of our ecosystem, and they serve many different roles. Their effects on our lives can be beneficial, harmful, or neutral. Harmful bacteria can cause milk to spoil and old vegetables or meats to decay. They can also cause a sore throat or a major debilitating disease, like tuberculosis or leprosy. The bacteria responsible for tuberculosis and leprosy are rod-shaped and are known as bacillus or bacilli (plural). The round or spherical bacteria are called cocci and these also include bacteria that can lead to sore throat (e.g. streptococcus pyogens) (Figure 4.1). We do have some useful bacteria that live in our food gut. These don't harm us and can help in food digestion. Another example of useful bacteria is *Staphylococcus lactis*. These bacteria are responsible for formation of yogurt from milk.

With so many bacteria around us, how do we recognize them? How do we distinguish one from another? Scientists have made various classifications, based upon different criteria. Bacteria can generally be divided into two main groups: eubacteria (in Greek *eu* means "good") or true bacteria, and archaebacteria (in Greek *archaios* means "ancient"). These two types of bacteria differ in many respects, including the composition of their membranes, the type of **ribosomes**, and structure of their **tRNA (transfer RNA)**. Most of the bacteria we encounter in our daily lives are eubacteria. For classification purposes, the kingdom of **prokaryotes** (organisms that lack a true membrane bound nucleus) is further divided. Bacteria are arranged into different classes, which are then subdivided into families.

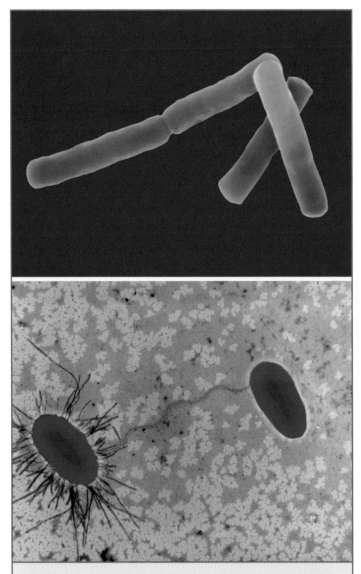

Figure 4.1 The bacteria that cause leprosy are rod shaped, such as the bacteria seen in this micrograph, taken with a scanning electron microscope and magnified 3,250 times (top). Bacteria can also be round in shape, such as the bacteria seen in the bottom picture (transmission electron microscope, magnified 5,000 times).

Each family has many genera, and each genus can have many species. As an example, *Mycobacteria* is a genus name. It belongs to the family *Mycobacteriaceae*. This family belongs to the class called *Actinomycetales*. The bacteria that causes leprosy is called *Mycobacterium leprae*, with *leprae* being the species name (Figure 4.2).

THE FAMILY OF *MYCOBACTERIA*

Many members of this group are free-living, but the group is probably best known for its animal pathogens. *M. bovis* causes tuberculosis in cattle, other ruminants, and primates. These pathogens can also cause diseases in humans, so cattle are tested routinely. The milk available for our consumption is generally pasteurized before sale. **Pasteurization** kills all harmful living pathogens, including *Mycobacteria* and prevents disease transmission. A close relative of *M. bovis* is *M. tuberculosis*, which causes tuberculosis in humans. *M. avium*, on the other hand, is associated with pneumonia in birds. Several other members of the family of mycrobacteria are known to be opportunist pathogens. They infect individuals who are weak, undernourished, or have weak immune systems. Many of these opportunist infections are found in AIDS patients.

Corynebacteria belong in the family *Mycobacteriaceae* and are part of the CMN group (*Corynebacteria*, *Mycobacteria*, and *Nocardia*). As a group, they produce long chain fatty acids called mycolic acids (discussed in Chapter 5). For *Corynebacteria*, chains of 28 to 40 carbons are common; for *Nocardia*, chains of 40 to 56 carbons are produced; for *Mycobacteria*, the chains are 60 to 90 carbons in length .

MYCOBACTERIUM LEPRAE

The *Mycobacterium leprae* bacillus, also known as Hansen's bacillus, ranges from 2 to 7 micrometers (1 micrometer =1/1000 of a millimeter) in length and 0.3 to 0.4 micrometers in width. Like many other bacteria, *M. leprae* has

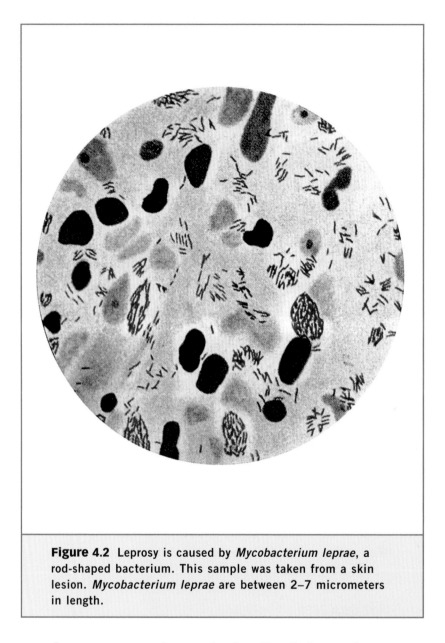

Figure 4.2 Leprosy is caused by *Mycobacterium leprae*, a rod-shaped bacterium. This sample was taken from a skin lesion. *Mycobacterium leprae* are between 2–7 micrometers in length.

four components: the capsule, the cell wall, the membrane, and the contents of the cell (cytoplasm and nucleic acid) (Figure 4.3). What makes it different from other bacteria is its unique cell wall or cell coat. These *Mycrobacteria* have a cell wall that is very rich in lipid (fats, oils) content, and they contain waxes. The complex fatty acids and lipid layer makes them **acid-fast**, or impenetrable to acids. The bacteria do not follow the normal bacterial staining principles and are resistant to treatment with an acid or alcohol. *M. leprae* stains with the Zeihl-Neelsen staining method, use carbol fuchsin, rather than with the traditional Gram staining method. The Zeihl-Neelsen staining method involves heating the bacterial smear on the slide with carbol fuchsin for about five minutes.

TUBERCULOSIS

In 1882, Robert Koch identified the organism that causes human tuberculosis (TB), *Mycobacterium tuberculosis*. At the time, TB was rampant, causing one-seventh of all deaths in Europe. Even today, the disease remains a global health problem, with around 1 billion people (over 20% of the world's population) infected worldwide. In the United States, the disease occurs most commonly among the elderly, malnourished people, alcoholics, impoverished males, and Native Americans. This bacterium is primarily transmitted through contact with the nasal or oral secretions of the infected patients.

Disease symptoms include fever, fatigue, and weight loss. The disease is generally characterized by a persistent cough. In many countries, individuals, especially infants, are vaccinated against this bacteria by BCG (Bacilli Calmette Guérin). The disease is preventable by maintaining better public health standards and improving social conditions, for example, reducing homelessness and drug abuse. Once someone is infected, the disease can be fully cured under supervised medical treatment, especially if detected in early stages.

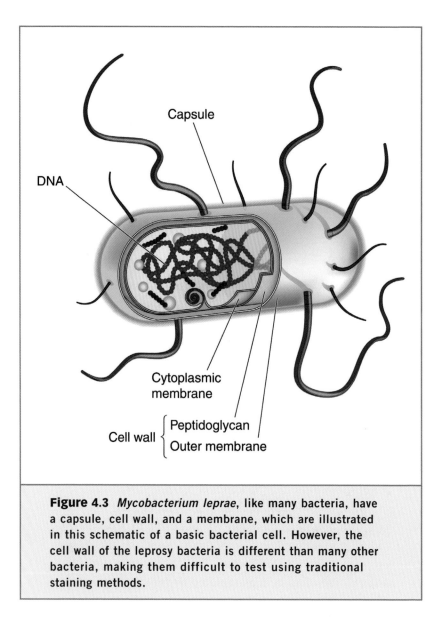

Figure 4.3 *Mycobacterium leprae*, like many bacteria, have a capsule, cell wall, and a membrane, which are illustrated in this schematic of a basic bacterial cell. However, the cell wall of the leprosy bacteria is different than many other bacteria, making them difficult to test using traditional staining methods.

THE CELL WALL

The bacterial cell wall is a semi-rigid, tight knit structure containing **peptidoglycan.** The main function for the cell wall is to prevent against **osmotic lysis.** These bacteria have a thick wax-coated cell wall. The major component of this cell wall is mycolic acid. In fact, it is the major component of the cell wall of the taxa actinomycetes. Different genera belonging to this class are *Mycobacterium, Gordona, Nocardia,* and *Rhodococcus.* Mycolic acids are localized in the inner leaflet of the cell wall, either covalently bound or loosely associated with polymers. These mycolic acids are complex hydroxylated branched-chain fatty acids, with 60 to 90 carbon molecules. Along with hydroxyl (-OH) groups, they can further diversify with different organic groups, like methoxy (CH_3O) and keto (CO).

In 1938, these fatty acids were first isolated from a waxy extract of human tubercle bacillus. Their common structure was revealed in 1950 by J. Asselineau. Now, mycolic acid forms a broad family of over 500 types. The mycolic acid from *Mycobacterium* can be more complex, with a range of functional groups, whereas other members may have simpler forms with no extra chemical groups. For classification purposes, the mycolic acids isolated from *Mycobacterium* are called eumycolic acids (or just mycolic acid). The acids isolated from *Corynebacterium* and *Nocardia* are named coryno-mycolic and nocardo-mycolic acids, respectively.

Mycolic acids are responsible for maintaining a rigid cell shape and may constitute up to 60% of the dry weight of an organism. They also make the bacteria resistant to chemical injury, thus protecting cells against hydrophobic (hydro=water, phobic= hate or fear) antibiotics (Isoniazid, which inhibits mycolic acid biosynthesis is an efficient antimycobacterial agent.) It is because of this waxy coating that the bacterium gains its hydrophobic characteristics. While this resistant cell wall continues to pose challenges in combating the microbe, **paleobiologists,** scientists who study the biology of fossil organism, have found a use for it. Because of the stable nature of the fatty acids, they can be used to identify the type and extent of disease found in ancient times. **Paleo-epidemiologists,** scientists who study disease in fossil organisms, can study fatty acids by analyzing the ancient skeletons.

WHERE IS THE LEPROSY BACILLUS FOUND?

The most natural and congenial environment for *M.leprae* is a eucaryotic cell, which, in most cases, is found in humans, but

HOW ARE BACTERIA COLORED?

Bacteria are among the smallest living organisms. They are single celled and vary in size from 0.5 micrometer (mm) to 10 mm (1mm=1/1000 cm). Imagine trying to see an object that is 100th the size of a sand particle. Because something so small cannot be seen with an unaided eye, scientists use microscopes. To make the visualization process easier and more informative, scientists have developed techniques to stain the bacteria, according to their composition, to help in their identification. The most common method used for bacterial staining is called Gram staining and was developed by the Danish physician Christian Gram in 1884.

In a microbiology lab, this simple staining method begins with applying bacteria to a slide. The slide is then soaked in a violet dye followed by iodine treatment. The slide is then rinsed with alcohol and counterstained with a pink dye called safranine. This staining procedure divides bacteria into two classes: gram-positive and gram-negative. The cell walls of gram-negative bacteria have a very low affinity for the violet stain, which is rinsed out by the alcohol. Once counterstained with safranine, however, the gram-negative bacteria appear bright pink or red. Gram-positive cell walls have a high affinity for the violet stain, and retain it, even through the alcohol rinse. When the process is complete, they appear dark purple or brown. The difference in composition of the bacterial cell walls leads to this differential staining. Gram-positive cell walls are about occasionally may be found in the nine-banded armadillo, the mouse footpad and, to a lesser degree, the monkey. Scientists have also been able to grow the majority of pathogenic *Mycobacteria* in a variety of laboratory culture media, with the help of various nutrients. *M. leprae* still cannot be cultivated artificially in laboratory media, causing much frustration and

five times as rich in peptidoglycan as gram-negative cell walls. Members of mycobacteria are unique in their cell wall composition and do not stain by this universal standard method. They are stained by a much harsher treatment that is also used in their identification (Figure 4.4).

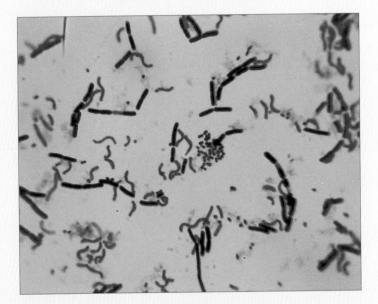

Figure 4.4 This micrograph (taken with a light microscope and magnified 1,000 times) shows both gram-positive and gram-negative bacteria. When stained with the Gram Stain technique, gram-positive bacteria appear purple and gram-negative bacteria appear pink or red.

delay in finding an effective anti-leprosy vaccine, or a thorough understanding of the bacteria.

The leprosy bacillus is an **obligate intracellular parasite**. It is a slow growing bacteria that multiplies with a generation time of 12.5 days. It grows best at 27–30°Celsius (80–86° Fahrenheit), hence its predilection for cooler areas of the human body (like finger tips).

5

Host-pathogen Interactions

Mycobacterium leprae attacks the host body as if it were a foreign invader. As a natural response to any such invasion, the host system tries to defend itself. First, it tries to prevent the invader from entering its system. Then, it tries to kill and eliminate the invader, once it is inside. This host response to pathogens is called the immune response. In short, the host tries to mount an immune response against the parasite, and the pathogen's natural reaction is to evade it. Before we talk more about the specific case of human response to *Mycobacterium*, let's look at a bit of general information about the immune system.

THE SYSTEM THAT PROTECTS US

The term *immunity* comes from the Latin expression *immunitas,* meaning "freedom from." Indeed, the immune system gives us freedom from the attack of innumerable pathogenic organisms and their ill effects. Every single organism needs some form of immunity, because every single form of organism can be attacked by another. Even bacteria have molecules that protect them from being hijacked by viruses. Bacteria, on the contrary, are very clever and keep trying to fool our immune system.

The ability of the immune system to mount a response to disease is dependent on many complex interactions between the components of the immune system and the antigens on the invading pathogens, or disease-causing agents. We will learn more about the cells of the immune system in the discussion that follows. Immunity in higher organisms, like vertebrates, can be divided into two major categories: innate and acquired.

INNATE IMMUNITY

The innate or natural immune system is that part of the immune system that we are born with. The innate immune system keeps out invading organisms (pathogens), such as viruses, bacteria, and fungi through a number of mechanisms. These mechanisms include physical barriers, such as the skin and the mucous layers; fever to overheat the invaders; pathogen destroying enzymes secreted in mucous layers and elsewhere; and acidic bodily secretions, which bacteria do not like. Other mechanisms through which the immune system keeps out invading bacteria include the complement—a system of plasma proteins that principally attack bacteria; the inflammatory response, which involves the action of several biochemicals and immune cells to destroy pathogens, prepare other cells to resist attack, and regulate downstream steps of the immune response; and nonspecific white blood cells, called effector cells, principally the **macrophages** that gobble up pathogens. Innate immunity is not specifically geared toward any particular kind of organism. It is a nonspecific array of defense mechanisms to prevent any organism from getting into or thriving in our systems.

ACQUIRED IMMUNITY

Also known as specific or adaptive immunity, acquired immunity focuses on those features of the immune system that are "learned" during a person's lifetime, rather than the immunity an individual is born with. This part of the immune system deals with specific invaders and learns to recognize them by exposure to them. Acquired immunity can function at different levels and in different forms, called humoral and cell-mediated immunity.

Humoral immunity principally operates through a type of white blood cell called a B-cell, which originates in bone marrow and the spleen. During humoral immune responses, proteins called antibodies, which can stick to and destroy **antigens** (any foreign molecule or organism which can elcit an immune response by our body), appear in the blood and other body fluids. These antibodies are produced specifically against each organism. Humoral immune responses resist invaders that act outside of cells, such as bacteria and toxins (poisonous substances produced by living organisms). Humoral immune responses can also prevent viruses from entering cells (Figure 5.1).

Cell-mediated immunity operates through another type of white blood cell called a T cell, which matures in the **thymus,** (a small glandular organ located behind the breast-bone). During cell-mediated immune responses, cells that can destroy other cells become active. Their destructive activity is limited to cells that are either infected with, or are producing, a specific antigen. The T cell system first recognizes some non-self molecules and then prepares its army against these invaders. With a new set of cells that have new tools (killer molecules), the T cells attack the infected body cells. For the T cells to recognize the infected cell as a target, the infected cell needs to look considerably different and display some new kind of molecular appearance, on their surface. Cell-mediated immune responses resist invaders that reproduce within the body cells, such as viruses. Cell-mediated responses may also destroy cells making mutated (changed) forms of normal molecules, as is the case in some cancers.

OTHER COMPONENTS OF THE IMMUNE SYSTEM
The immune system is very complex and there are some more terms we need to understand before we understand how "smart" the leprosy bacillus is.

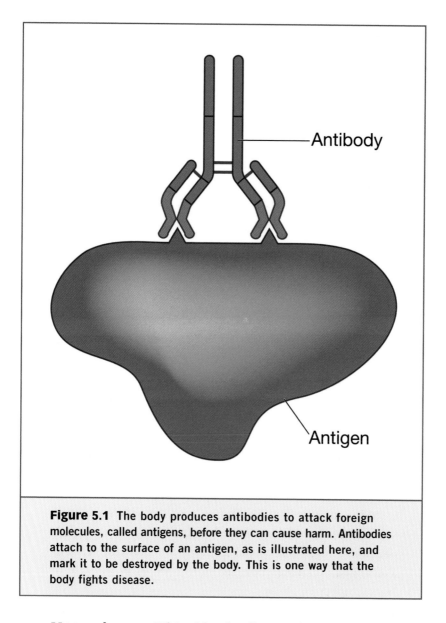

Figure 5.1 The body produces antibodies to attack foreign molecules, called antigens, before they can cause harm. Antibodies attach to the surface of an antigen, as is illustrated here, and mark it to be destroyed by the body. This is one way that the body fights disease.

Macrophages: White blood cells are the mainstay of the immune system. Some white blood cells, known as macrophages, play a function in innate immunity by surrounding, ingesting, and destroying invading bacteria and other foreign organisms in a process called **phagocytosis** (literally, "cell eating"), which is part of the inflammatory reaction. Macrophages also play an important role in adaptive immunity in that they attach to invading antigens and deliver them to be destroyed by other components of the adaptive immune system (Figure 5.2).

Lymphocytes: Lymphocytes are specialized white blood cells whose function is to identify and destroy invading antigens. All lymphocytes begin as "stem cells" in the bone marrow, the soft tissue that fills most bone cavities, but they mature in two different places. Some lymphocytes mature in the bone marrow and are called B lymphocytes. B lymphocytes, or B cells, make antibodies, which circulate through the blood and other body fluids, binding to antigens and helping to destroy them in humoral immune responses.

Other lymphocytes, called T lymphocytes, or T cells, mature in the thymus (as described in the previous section). Some T lymphocytes, called **cytotoxic** (cell-poisoning) or killer T lymphocytes, generate cell-mediated immune responses, directly destroying cells that have specific antigens on their surface, which are recognized by the killer T cells. Helper T lymphocytes, a second kind of T lymphocyte, regulate the immune system by controlling the strength and quality of all immune responses.

Most contact between antigens and lymphocytes occurs in the lymphoid organs—the lymph nodes, spleen, and tonsils, as well as in specialized areas of the intestines and lungs. Mature lymphocytes constantly travel through the blood to the lymphoid organs and then back to the blood again. This recirculation ensures that the body is continuously monitored for invading substances.

Antigen receptors: One of the characteristics of adaptive immunity is that it is specific. Each response is tailored to a

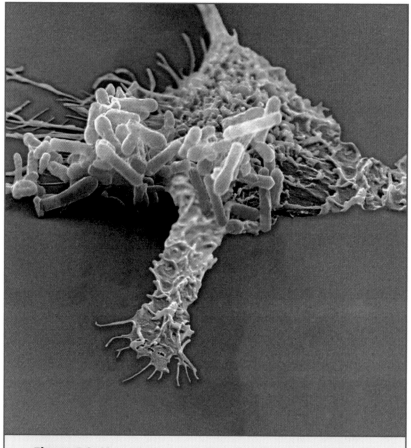

Figure 5.2 Macrophages are a type of white blood cell that destroy foreign invaders by swallowing them. The macrophage in this picture has extended "arms" around the rod-shaped bacteria and is attempting to clear the bacteria from the organism's body before they can cause harm.

specific type of invading antigen. Each lymphocyte, as it matures, makes an **antigen receptor**—that is, a specific structure on its surface that can bind with a matching structure on the antigen like a lock and key. Although lymphocytes can make billions of different kinds of antigen receptors, each individual lymphocyte makes only one kind of receptor. When an antigen enters the body, it activates only the lymphocytes whose receptors match up with it.

Antigen presenting cells: When an antigen enters a cell, certain transport molecules within the cell attach themselves to the antigen and transport it to the surface of the cell, where they "present" the antigen to T lymphocytes. These transport molecules are made by a group of genes called the **major histo-compatibility complex (MHC)** and are therefore known as MHC molecules. Some MHC molecules, called class I MHC molecules, present antigens to killer T cells; other MHC molecules, called class II MHC molecules, present antigens to helper T cells.

FAVORITE TARGETS OF *M. LEPRAE*

Most pathogens prefer one kind of cell in our system to another. Not all cells are the same. Not all of them provide the best environment or food to the invading pathogen. The *M. leprae* bacterium invades peripheral nerves and skin cells and becomes an obligate intracellular parasite—that is, it is a parasite that can live only in this environment. It is most frequently found in the Schwann cells and mono nuclear phagocytes (macrophages). The *M. leprae* shows a strong affinity toward a protein called **laminin,** which is specifically found in nerve tissues. That partially explains its affinity toward Schwann cells. Macrophages are described as the part of the "components of the immune system."

WHAT HAPPENS WHEN *M. LEPRAE*
AND OUR BODY SEE EACH OTHER?

Because living *M. leprae* produce no toxins and no power of locomotion, it is thought that they cannot enter unbroken skin or intact mucous membranes. This issue, however, is still the source of much debate. Most **leprologists** believe that *M. leprae* can only enter through a break in the skin, and through the mucous membrane of the nose, in particular.

After *M.leprae* gain entry into the body, they can provoke one of three possible, responses, contingent upon the measure of cell-mediated immunity (CMI) in the host. To begin with, they could be ingested by the macrophages and completely digested, if CMI is present. This action can take place at the point of entry or at the lymph nodes to where they may be transported inside the large defense cells (macrophages). This type of action is believed to take place in most people infected by *M.leprae*, many of whom may never know they have been invaded by the leprosy bacilli. Approximately 90 to 95% of people exposed to leprosy experience this defensive action of the body.

Second, in persons with no resistance (lack of CMI), *M.leprae* freely multiply, even within the very cells (macrophage) that

SCHWANN CELLS

Various support cells are associated with neurons, most typically, Schwann cells. A neuron is made up of a dendrite that receives the impulse (from another nerve cell or from a sensory organ), the cell body (numbers of which side-by-side form gray matter) where the nucleus is found, and the axon which carries the impulse away from the cell. Wrapped around the axon are the Schwann cells, and the spaces/junctions between Schwann cells are called nodes of Ranvier. Collectively, the Schwann cells make up the myelin sheath (numbers of which side-by-side form white matter). Schwann cells wrap around the axon. Having an intact myelin sheath and nodes of Ranvier are critical to proper travel of the nerve impulse. Diseases that destroy the myelin sheath (demyelinating disorders) can cause paralysis or other problems. Schwann cells are analogous to the insulation on electrical wires, and just as electrical wires short out if there's a problem with the insulation, so too, can neurons malfunction when myelin sheaths are not intact (Figure 5.3).

are meant to destroy them. It is not uncommon for up to 300 *M. leprae* to proliferate inside these large defense cells, which later transport the multiplying and dying (of old age) bacilli from the site of entry to many different parts of the body. This multiplication of the bacilli, even in the defense cells, is the most serious—and contagious—form of leprosy, known as lepromatous or multibacilliary (MB) leprosy.

Third, some patients have some resistance to the infecting bacilli, but not enough immunity to completely destroy the organisms. Their defense system allows a limited, but variable, multiplication of the bacilli, contingent upon the degree of CMI. In some patients—those with the tuberculoid form of the disease—many of the bacilli are killed off by the body's defenses, which keep the infection localized to a small area of

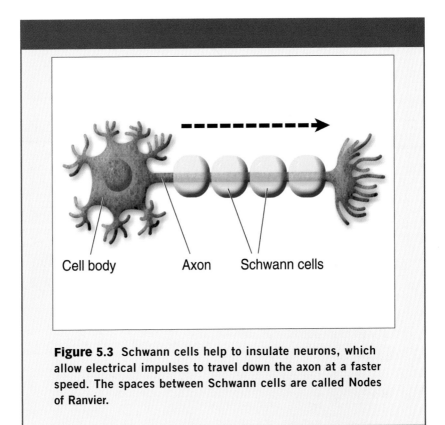

Cell body Axon Schwann cells

Figure 5.3 Schwann cells help to insulate neurons, which allow electrical impulses to travel down the axon at a faster speed. The spaces between Schwann cells are called Nodes of Ranvier.

the body. In other patients, with a lesser degree of immunity, the disease may be somewhat generalized, with leprosy lesions scattered in different places. This form of the disease falls in the "borderline" category. Borderline leprosy is immunologically unstable.

These groups constitute what is called the immunological spectrum, ranging from those with a strong CMI at the tuberculoid end, to the more serious types, with a CMI deficit at the lepromatous or infectious end. There is another group, which is not considered as part of the spectrum. In its early stage, it is not known whether it will progress into the spectrum to become tuberculoid or lepromatous, so it is known as the indeterminate form of the disease.

DAMAGE CAUSED BY INFECTION

The pathology associated with the disease is due to the body's immune response, rather than direct damage caused by the bacteria. Most reactions are mainly observed during or after multi-drug treatment (MDT). Leprosy reactions typically represent acute inflammatory episodes of two major kinds: erythema nodosum leprosum (ENL) or type II leprosy reactions, and reversal reactions (RR) or type I reaction. ENL occurs in patients with lepromatous leprosy and RR is seen in patients with borderline leprosy. Lepromatous leprosy is characterized by the absence of specific cellular immunity. Therefore, there is uncontrolled proliferation of the bacilii with many lesions and extensive infiltration of the skin and the nerves. The dermis contains foamy macrophages filled with many bacteria, but few mature T lymphocytes. Tuberculoid leprosy patients have a vigorous cellular immune response to the *Mycobacterium*, which limits the disease to a few well-defined skin patches or nerve trunks. This type of reaction generally leads to severe nerve damage.

Bacteria can directly or indirectly induce cell death or **apoptosis** of the host Schwann cells. The presence of bacterial proteins in the nerve cell is recognized by the immune system. Our cell-mediated immune system, involving T cells, tries to rapidly detect invading pathogens and get rid of them, causing the Schwann cells harboring the bacteria to be identified and eliminated from the system. This causes removal of the important nerve cells and debilitating neural damage. This process also destroys nerve cells close to the infected Schwann cells, resulting in large-scale nerve damage. Technically speaking, reversal reactions are the primary cause of nerve damage.

6

Controlling the Disease

When we experience physical discomfort, we are often told to see a physician. But how does the physician know what is causing our pain and how to cure it? Medical science has made many advances over the years, and now has certain ways of assigning a symptom to a causative agent or a known medical condition. This process is known as diagnosing a disease or condition. Each ailment will have its own characteristic hallmarks or symptoms, which distinguish it from other diseases. However, many signs can be shared among several conditions—like fever, headache, and fatigue. Medical science often plays a very important role in correctly diagnosing an ailment and then treating the patient appropriately.

HOW IS LEPROSY DIAGNOSED?

Given the severely debilitating form the disease can take, early diagnosis is essential. Unfortunately, this disease can superficially mimic many dermatological and neurological conditions. The first signs of the disease start with discoloration (change in normal color) of the skin. Certain spots on the skin can become darker **(hyperpigmented)** or lighter (hypopigmented). These spots also become anaesthetic (loose sense of touch, heat, cold or pain). Such spots can appear anywhere on the body and should be immediately reported to a physician. Other signs of the disease include thickening of nerves and lesions in mucous membranes (like in the nose). Anaesthetic skin or mucous membrane lesions in the presence of enlarged nerves are also hallmarks of the disease. Primary diagnosis is confirmed by taking samples from the skin. Smear **biopsies** (small pieces of tissue) are taken from the skin and then stained to detect bacteria. The density of bacteria observed is recorded logarithmically, as the bacterial index (BI). Although this test can confirm the presence of the disease, it does have a limitation. If the amount of bacteria is too low, they will not show up in the test.

In addition to microscopic detection, other methods are used, as well. The most widely used serological test works by detecting antibodies against the phenolic glycolipid-1 (PGL-1). Antibodies are produced by our body against the bacterial proteins, if there is an infection. These tests also have a limitation. They can identify 90% of the severely infective or lepromatous form of the disease, but only 40 to 50% of mildly infective or paucibacillary patients.[12] Such antibodies are also found in 1 to 5% of healthy individuals living in infected areas. Diagnosis using polymerase chain reaction (PCR) also has similar limitations. It can diagnose 97% of multibacillary patients, but only 44% of paucibacillary patients.[13] PCR is only useful clinically to support a diagnosis of leprosy when atypical signs or characteristics are present. It was used to detect the spread of disease in ancient times, as discussed in Chapter 3. Ultimately, effective diagnosis in a person with very low bacterial loads is still a challenge.

DRUG DEVELOPMENT

As we learned in Chapter 1, devising a proper curative treatment for leprosy took time. Over many decades, and through lots of trial and error, scientists eventually reached a situation of greater confidence. Further study, in order to promote greater understanding, is still ongoing, however.

Toward the end of 19th century (as is still true today), this disease was still affecting more human lives in India than anywhere else in the world. Initial attempts at drug therapy were the result of early information about herbal therapy. Meanwhile, research continued to improve on the chaulmoogra oil treatment, which was anything but the ideal therapy. Taken orally, it produced nausea, while injections of the thick oil were quite painful. In 1937, after a distinguished career, Wellesley Bailey died, but not before seeing real hope for the patients he had come to love and serve. Hope came in the form of the discovery of one of the most revolutionary drugs of its day. As early at 1908, German Chemist Gerhardt Domack had made successful attempts to produce what eventually became the parent chemical in the sulphone family of drugs. Out of this research, evolved diamino diphenyl sulphone, (Dapsone, or DDS), although at the time, no one associated DDS with a possible cure for leprosy. It was considered too toxic a drug to be used on humans. In 1941, American physician Dr. Faget was courageous enough to use the parent sulphone drug, with encouraging results (Figure 6.1).

Even then, as a bacteriostatic drug, DDS did not actually kill the leprosy bacilli. It only prevented their multiplication. For many years, it did seem that Dapsone would eventually help in eliminating leprosy—that is, until resistant organisms began to appear. Fortunately, new and more potent drugs, such as Rifampicin, became available. Rifampicin, in combination with other drugs (multi-drug therapy, or MDT), has given real hope that, sometime in the future, the elimination of leprosy could possibly become a reality. Rifampicin also kills the very well-known cousin of *M. leprae*, *M. tuberculosis*. This drug acts by stopping the synthesis of messenger RNA from DNA, by affecting the enzyme (RNA polymerase) important for this process (Figure 6.2). Rifampicin is specific to the bacterial enzyme, and does not harm our enzyme function.

In 1981, the World Health Organization started recommending multi-drug therapy. Three drugs are taken in combination: Dapsone, Rifampicin (or Rifampin), and Clofazimine. Treatment takes anywhere from six months to a year or more, depending on the extent and character of the disease. Multi-drug treatment has brought new hope to millions of leprosy patients, and, combined with more efficient means of diagnosis, has resulted in the prevention of ulceration, crippling deformities, and other disabilities. Multi-drug treatment helps to ensure that a drug-resistant form of the leprosy bacterium will not develop.

NEW LEPROSY DRUG

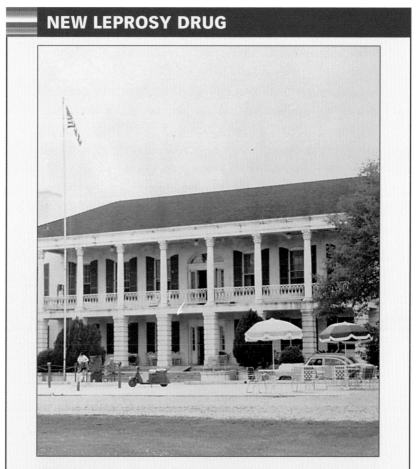

Figure 6.1 In 1941, Dr. Guy Faget began administering the first successful treatment for leprosy at the Carville Research Center in Carville, Louisiana (shown above). The new sulfone drug, Promin, proved successful in rendering leprosy patients non-infectious. Today, several drugs are used in a multi-drug fashion for 6 to 24 months to treat the disease.

In addition, intensive health educational programs have helped alleviate the misunderstandings and social stigma often associated with the disease.

Leprosy treatment is not perfect, however. It can cause severe side effects. These side effects are not the result of the drugs themselves, but come instead as a result of inflammation that develops when large numbers of leprosy bacteria are killed and broken down inside the body. Freeing the body of dead organisms is essential and can be accomplished by administering additional drugs to the patient. The inflammation must be treated with anti-inflammatory drugs, such as corticosteroids, to minimize additional nerve damage. Aspirin and prednisone can also control inflammation, generally known as "erythema nodosum leprosum" (ENL), which may occur with therapy. Inflammation can cause fever, skin lesions, and other symptoms, which are thought to be a result of abnormal immune reactions, against the killed bacteria (as they are still foreign to our body).

Since the 1970s, studies have shown that ENL can be effectively treated with the controversial drug known as thalidomide. This drug does not attack the leprosy bacteria directly, but helps to relieve the inflammation and heal the skin sores in patients with ENL. In July 1998, the Food and Drug Administration (FDA) approved thalidomide for the treatment of ENL. The approval of thalidomide has been queen controversial, however. In the early 1960s, the drug was found to cause severe birth defects in thousands of babies born in Europe, where thalidomide was often prescribed for pregnant women suffering from morning sickness (Figure 6.3). The drug, which was never approved in the United States, was banned from pharmacies after it was linked to more than 10,000 infants born with shortened, flipper-like limbs and other serious deformities.[14]

Leprosy can be avoided by covering the face and hands when in the presence of infected individuals, and modern

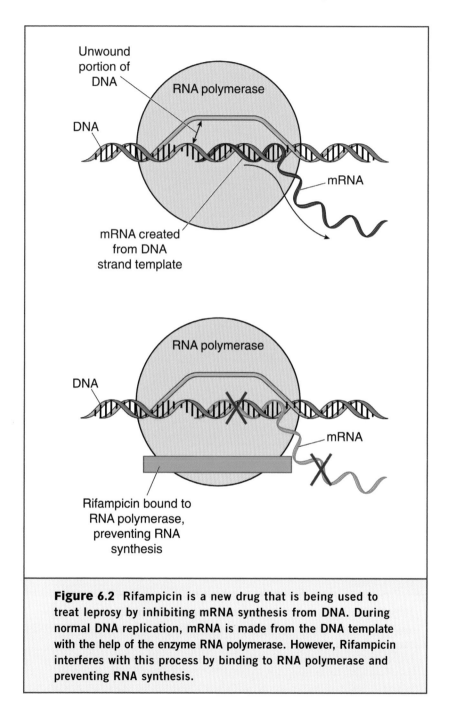

Figure 6.2 Rifampicin is a new drug that is being used to treat leprosy by inhibiting mRNA synthesis from DNA. During normal DNA replication, mRNA is made from the DNA template with the help of the enzyme RNA polymerase. However, Rifampicin interferes with this process by binding to RNA polymerase and preventing RNA synthesis.

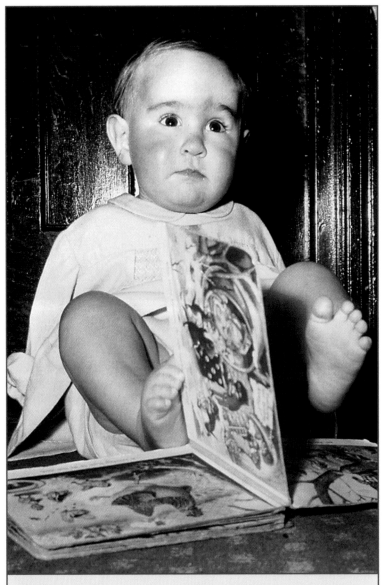

Figure 6.3 ENL, or erythema nodosum leprosum, can be treated with the drug thalidomide. However, thalidomide is dangerous for pregnant women, as it can cause severe birth defects such as shortened or absent arms and legs. The baby in this picture suffers from the effects of thalidomide.

antibiotics and new treatment regimens are helping to keep the number of severely disfigured individuals to a minimum. Killing bacilli *(M. leprae)* by multi-drug therapy is only one measure of successful treatment for leprosy. Nerve damage, leprosy's hallmark symptom, is not reversed by MDT, however. Many treated patients still need rehabilitation, while others suffer from the enormous psychological stigma of the disease.

7

Understanding the
M. leprae Bacillus

Undoubtedly, for scientists to better understand a pathogen, that pathogen needs to exist in large enough number to be studied. In essence, scientists must understand the full strength of the "enemy," before making any attempt to manipulate it. Unfortunately, scientists are still struggling with the leprosy bacillus, in this regard.

Most bacteria can normally be grown in a laboratory, in an artificial setting. Free-living and non-pathogenic bacteria are easy to cultivate, and can be grown in relatively simple media. This type of bacteria can metabolize a mixture of protein, salt, and carbohydrates in order to grow. They have all the metabolic pathways and enzymes to grow from basic substrates. In fact, the ease of growing some of these bacteria and the ability to manipulate them has provided biologists with a very useful tool. The most commonly used bacteria in biological laboratories is a gram-negative bacillus called *Escherichia coli*.

Unfortunately, growing pathogenic bacteria is not as easy. Many parasitic bacteria need specialized medium to grow and divide. Examples include blood agar, which is used to grow *Lactococcus pneumoniae*, *Staphylococcus aureus*; and chocolate agar, which is used to culture *Haemophilus influenzae* and *Neisseria gonorrhoeae*. Growing different species of *Mycobacteria* has long been a challenge. Whereas some species of *Mycobacteria*, like *M. tuberculosis* and *M. bovis* can be grown *in vitro*, under special conditions, *M. leprae* has never been grown in artificial media. It is an obligate intracellular pathogen, which means that it can grow only inside a living cell and can never exist freely by itself. Because the bacteria refuse to grow artificially, scientists must find another way to study it.

Of course, one way to accomplish this is to isolate bacteria from the patients and then use them for experiments.

E. coli

Escherichia coli (*E. coli*, for short) is a bacterium that normally lives in the intestines of humans and other animals. Most types of *E. coli* are harmless, but some can cause disease. Disease-causing *E. coli* are grouped according to the different ways by which they cause illness. Enterotoxigenic *Escherichia coli*, or ETEC, is the name given to a group of *E. coli* that produce special toxins which stimulate the lining of the intestines causing them to secrete excessive fluid, thus producing diarrhea.

The organism can be found on a small number of cattle farms and can live in the intestines of healthy cattle. Meat can become contaminated during slaughter, and organisms can be thoroughly mixed into beef when it is ground. Bacteria present on the cow's udders or on equipment may get into raw milk.

Eating meat, especially ground beef, which has not been cooked sufficiently to kill *E. coli,* can cause infection. Contaminated meat looks and smells normal. Although the number of organisms required to cause disease is not known, it is suspected to be very small. Among other known sources of infection are consumption of sprouts, lettuce, salami, unpasteurized milk and juice, and swimming in or drinking sewage-contaminated water.

Bacteria in diarrheal stools of infected persons can be passed from one person to another if hygiene or hand washing habits are inadequate. This is particularly likely among toddlers who are not toilet trained. Family members and playmates of these children are at high risk of becoming infected.

Although this approach is used for many experiments, the number of bacteria available is limited, and very few studies can be conducted. In addition, complications such as finding patients and taking split-skin smears make this method impractical. Further, there is also a chance of isolating multiple types of bacteria from the same patient, thus negatively affecting the results. Another method of experimentation involves using some other animals as a host for the *M. leprae* bacillus.

To a large extent, humans have been the only naturally occurring host known for *M. leprae*, but that has changed. Armadillos (*Dasypus novemcintus*) can also become infected with the leprosy bacteria. This useful discovery allowed scientists to bring armadillos into their laboratories to inject them with the bacteria. The injected bacteria could cause the disease and, at times, produce faster and more severe symptoms than seen in humans. This realization provided the researchers with a constant supply of bacteria to be used for many more experiments.

In addition to armadillos, scientists have had some success growing the bacteria in mouse footpads. Still, culturing them takes a long time, as the bacteria divide very slowly, around once every 15 to 20 days.

ARMADILLOS: THE ANIMAL OF CHOICE

Armadillos are not commonly used to grow the leprosy bacteria, but, in addition to being able to grow the bacteria, they also have other advantages. They are the only mammals known to routinely give birth to quadruplets. Sometimes, embryos die and triplets or twins are born, but the standard litter size for armadillos is generally four identical pups. Derived from single fertilized ovum, all four are the same sex and all contain identical sets of genes, a major advantage for scientists seeking to learn whether genetic predisposition plays a part in the transmission of leprosy. No concrete documentation exists to link leprosy with any particular genetic makeup, but these studies will be very informative. In addition, the armadillo quadruplets are good test and control subjects for any experiment. These football-sized mammals are tolerant of laboratory procedures, unlikely to bite, and a have a large population, with about 30 million in the United States alone (Figure 7.1).

The use of armadillos infected with leprosy has enabled researchers to search for new drugs and to test whether older drugs induce resistance after prolonged treatment. Similarly, vaccine attempts depend upon the bacteria grown and isolated from artificially infected armadillos.

THE AMAZING ARMADILLOS

The nine-banded armadillo, found in northern Argentina and the southern United States, and a few close armadillo cousins are found in South America. In general, armadillos are well liked—and amusing. Homely, ungainly, and not too bright, they epitomize the underdog and elicit our sympathy. Armadillo festivals, races, comic books, T-shirts, and posters have swept the South during the past decade. Texas jewelers have recently advertised gold armadillo rings, pendants, and pins. Many people eat armadillos and they are considered a delicacy in parts of Mexico.

All armadillos in the United States vanished between 5,000 and 10,000 years ago, for unknown reasons. The many thousands of nine-banded armadillos that now exist in Florida are probably descendants of a fecund few that escaped from captivity near Cocoa, Florida, only half a century ago. The immigrant nine-banded armadillos from South America did survive in Mexico, and from there, during the 19th century, began one of the most rapid expansions in mammalian history. They were first reported in southern Texas in 1854. Blocked by the western deserts, they spread north to Kansas and Missouri and east toward Florida.

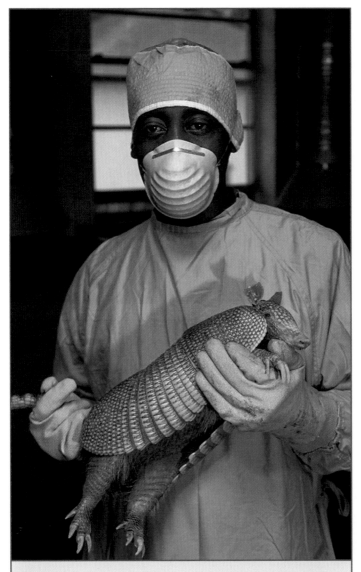

Figure 7.1 Armadillos are used for leprosy research. They are suitable hosts to grow the leprosy bacteria and monitor the disease. The hope is that by using armadillos as models, scientists can find better and more effective treatments for leprosy. The researcher in this picture holds an armadillo at the Carville Leprosy Clinic in Carville, Louisiana.

Of all the animals in the world, why would armadillos be the preferred hosts for leprosy? From the previous chapters, we know that the leprosy bacillus likes to stay in the cooler parts of the body (nose, ears, finger tips, toes, scrotum). The armadillo's body temperature ranges from between 28 to 33° C (82.4 to 91.4° F) compared to 37° C (98.6° F) for humans.[15] Leprosy bacteria undoubtedly feel "at home" in armadillos. Armadillos can live for 12 to 15 years in captivity, providing ample time to develop advanced disease symptoms. It is interesting to note that mouse footpads also have a lower temperature and are cooler, thus also serving as a suitable habitat for *M. leprae*.

Armadillos in the wild can have leprosy, which creates a concern about the ability of the disease spreading to people. Thus far, however, very little evidence exists to suggest that the disease can be transmitted in nature from armadillos to humans. Although the hypothetical possibility of an endemic always exists, the chances of it occurring are meager, at best.

GENOME SEQUENCING

We owe a lot to armadillos, with respect to our understanding of the bacteria that causes leprosy. All organisms remain a mystery, until we have deciphered their genes and functions, at international levels, with help from many different groups, scientists, and institutions. Scientists want to know about all of the genes an organism has. This is achieved by **genomic sequencing** (sequencing all DNA) from any organism in question. **Bioinformatics,** the application of computer science to the interpretation and management of biological data, has provided many software programs and databases, which help in quick, informative analyses of the obtained sequences. It is important to know the DNA sequence, as the DNA holds all the information about an organism—what it is, how it works, and how it behaves.

Scientists have made a similar attempt to sequence *M. leprae*. The bacteria for such a vast project were obtained from an armadillo-derived Indian isolate. The bacteria used was isolated from India and grown in armadillos. The leprosy bacterium has 3.27 Mb (mega base pair) genomes that have been mapped. This genome size is much smaller than that of its close relative *M. tuberculosis*, which has a genome size of 4.4 Mb. The genomic sequence revealed many other differences between the two species. *M. leprae* has only 1,600 genes, compared with 4,000 genes in *M. tuberculosis*.[16] The rest of the genome appears to be cluttered with more than 1,100 **pseudogenes**, which resemble genes in *M. tuberculosis*, but are no longer active. One clear conclusion from these results is that the *M. leprae* genome is severely contracted (Figure 7.2). The bacteria have lost many genes involved in metabolic pathways and many enzymes. This massive gene decay is unprecedented in sequenced genomes and likely explains why the leprosy bacillus is so resistant to artificial culture. It might also provide a reason for the unusually long division time for the bacteria.

Scientists have made some progress in understanding the interaction of these bacteria with their preferred host cells— Schwann cells. Schwann cells are present in the peripheral

HOW DO BACTERIA LOOK IN THE LAB?

Bacteria are grown on solid media that contain peptone, yeast extract, and sodium chloride (yes, even bacteria like common table salt). These components are mixed in water and then agar is added to solidify the media. After mixing all these things together, the mixture is **autoclaved** (boiled under high pressure to kill all living organisms). Then, the media is ready. It is poured into dishes, allowed to set, and used for growing bacteria. Starting from a very small number of bacteria, it normally takes 12 to 16 hours to get a plate full of laboratory bacteria. Unfortunately, things don't work that fast for the pathogenic bacteria.

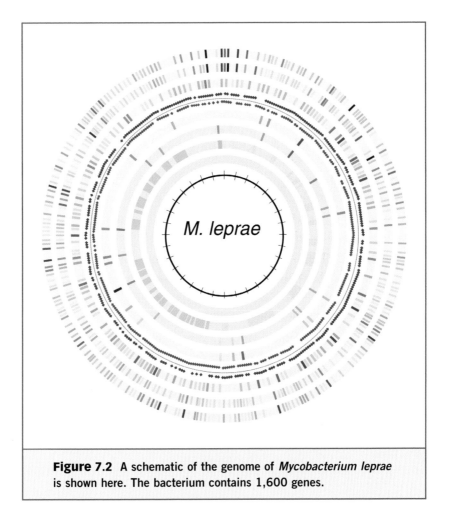

Figure 7.2 A schematic of the genome of *Mycobacterium leprae* is shown here. The bacterium contains 1,600 genes.

nervous system and help to separate and insulate nerve cells. Recent advances in culture techniques of Schwann cells and Schwann cell/axon cultures have given rise to detailed investigations of *M. leprae* Schwann cell interactions *in vitro*. These studies may one day provide scientists with vaccine molecules that help protect humans from leprosy.

8

Ongoing Reforms and the Future

HAS THE SOCIAL STIGMA CHANGED?

Scientifically, leprosy is an infectious disease that can affect anyone. The disease does not discriminate and is not a reflection of a patient's moral values or past sins. Unfortunately, this message is still not widely accepted or understood. Like many other issues, education and empathy are required in accepting leprosy-infected people into society. Many people living in remote areas are still not able to accept patients back into their lives. Most of those affected by the disease lead a normal healthy life after treatment and do not pose a risk of transmitting the disease any further. If, however, the infection has caused them any physical deformity or disfigurement, patients can have a tough time fitting in with their families and friends.

On the border of India and Nepal, leprosy patients who had been shunned from society gathered together and made their living mainly by begging. Their fate began to change in 1981, however, when reform efforts in the name of The Little Flower Institution were started by Baba Christdas. Little Flower is an institute for treating people with leprosy, helping them to lead normal lives and earn an independent living. The colony began with a hospital and doctors, for treatments. With time and financial support, it now owns a cattle dairy and has a cotton-based handloom industry where patients can work. When this effort was initiated, the milk and textile products produced by Little Flower had a tough time finding a market. Now, with increased public awareness, the dairy producers can barely keep up with the market demand, allowing patients to recover from the disease and live with dignity and respect. Many of these patients, however, come from poor, uneducated families and societies, where they will have a difficult time being accepted. The institute continues helping patients with the following message: "Leprosy is a poor man's disease, treat the patients like other human beings."[17]

DIFFERENT WORLDWIDE EFFORTS

Leprosy is being managed at the global level by the World Health Organization. In addition, various efforts at the individual country level aim to curb the disease within given political boundaries. The Indian Council for Medical Research (ICMR) has many institutions dedicated to the study of leprosy, from an epidemiological and drug discovery perspective. KIT Biomedical Research Center in the Netherlands serves as a knowledge center, giving advice to researchers, policy makers, and health workers all over the world. The National Institute of Health (NIH) has various research programs supporting leprosy research in the United States. Similarly, there are institutions in Nigeria (Leprosy Research Unit, eastern Nigeria), and in Yemen (Yemen Leprosy Elimination Society). In Brazil, the government has initiated an improved health program. They have also started to educate the public through the media, in an effort to decrease the social stigma associated with leprosy (Figure 8.1).

In addition, the International Leprosy Elimination Program (ILEP) promotes and facilitates cooperation between its members by coordinating the different leprosy programs, providing technical expertise, and representing the common interests. ILEP is an international federation of different, autonomous, nongovernment anti-leprosy organizations.

IS A VACCINE A POSSIBILITY?

During an invasion by a foreign organism, the body's defense mechanisms become quite active as they attempt to evade the

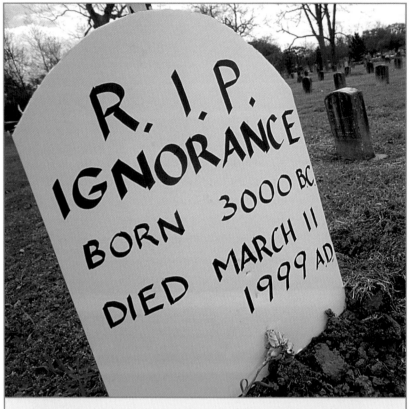

Figure 8.1 Research and education helps to reduce, and even eliminate, ignorance about leprosy. This sign, placed in the Gillis W. Long Hansen's Disease Center cemetery, shows that education leads to acceptance.

attack and protect the body from becoming ill. It is important to remember that the host-parasite relationship is a naturally occurring and continuously evolving phenomenon. For every defense that our body builds, parasites try to overcome it with a modified strategy. It becomes important to artificially intervene in this cycle, to prevent humans from further infection. These interventions can function at two levels: prevention or cure. A disease can be cured by killing the pathogen that caused it, and by healing the damages caused by the invader.

Another approach involves preventing the disease from occurring in the first place. This is achieved by boosting the body's immune response, and preparing it against any future infections. Successful vaccine candidates can be dead or inactive pathogens (like the vaccines against polio and smallpox) or part of the pathogen. There are vaccines available for bacterial diseases like diphtheria, tetanus, pertussis (whooping cough), tuberculosis, and typhoid fever. The BCG vaccine that is used for tuberculosis has also been tried for leprosy. It has been reported to be partially effective against the disease. A worldwide BCG vaccination program against *M. leprae* is not economically feasible, however. There have been some other vaccine trials using different combinations of heat-killed *M. leprae* and BCG, with some *Mycobacterium* isolates that can be grown in the laboratory. Results of these studies have been mixed, however, and not absolutely protective. In the absence of a successful vaccine candidate, MDT remains the only adequate weapon against *M. leprae*.

WHAT IS THE WORLD HEALTH ORGANIZATION?

The World Health Organization (WHO) is the United Nations' specialized agency for health. Established in 1948, the WHO's mission is the attainment of the highest possible level of health for all people worldwide. Health, as defined by the WHO, is a state of complete physical, mental, and social well-being, and not merely the absence of disease or infirmity.

The WHO is governed by 192 member states through the World Health Assembly. The Health Assembly is composed of representatives from the WHO's member states. The WHO member states are grouped into six regions, each with its own regional office.

Efforts are underway to find the bacterial components (cell wall and bacterial membrane) that can elicit a strong immune response in the body, to keep it prepared to fight any future attack. Such components can serve as successful vaccines.

Leprosy has been largely eradicated from Europe, North America, and Japan, as living conditions have improved for the general population and as potable water, sanitation, and adequate nutrition have become accessible to people in all social classes. Global attempts are underway to eliminate the leprosy bacteria. The slow growth of the pathogen, the apparent lack of environmental or animal reservoirs, low infectivity, and availability of effective therapy make it an ideal target for elimination.

NEW DRUGS AND THE FUTURE

Multi-drug therapy, which is currently in use, has proven the most effective way to fight this disease. The search for new drugs, however, continues. An attempt to identify drugs that can stop the neural damage caused by the bacteria will be a great help. Bacteria recognize certain molecules on the host cells' surface, which helps in binding. After identifying the right target cell, the bacteria bind to some proteins and enter a new home. Attempts are underway to understand the host cell molecules that may help in bacterial entry. Some host cell proteins, like dystroglycan, belonging to the family of glyco-proteins, have already been identified as potential binding molecules. Any drug that can prevent binding of the bacteria to these host molecules will prevent entry of bacteria into the nerve cell, stopping any subsequent neural damage.

Researchers are working to find more host proteins, which are essential for the bacterial infection in our bodies. The ultimate goal is to find new targets for drugs. In addition, the continuous hunt for new drug targets can provide backup, in the event the bacteria develop drug resistance to the existing mechanisms.

Nerve damage and the resulting disabilities are the major cause of **morbidity** among leprosy patients. These damages can cripple a patient for the rest of their lives, even after being cured of the disease. Different preventive procedures (management of reactions, nerve decompression) and corrective procedures (tendon transfers, management of plantar ulcers) are available to manage deformities. In addition, the availability of surgery, timely physiotherapy, and health education are very important in the prevention, management, and rehabilitation resulting from the disabilities associated with the disease. As leprosy patients continue to experience disabilities, these services will continue to be required. Compassion has never been more necessary than it is in the fight against this disease.

Glossary

Acid fast staining—A staining procedure that differentiates between bacteria, based on their ability to retain a dye when washed with an acid-alcohol solution.

Anaesthetic—Unable to sense touch, heat, cold, or pain.

Antigens—Any foreign particle that, upon entering our body, can cause an immune response.

Antigen receptor—Protein molecules that look similar to antibodies, found on the surface of specialized immune cells.

AIDS (acquired immune deficiency syndrome)—A disease caused by the HIV virus.

Apoptosis—Programmed cell death; normal process in which cells perish in an orderly, highly controlled manner in order to sculpt and control an organism's development.

Autoclave—An apparatus for sterilizing objects through the use of steam under pressure.

Bioinformatics—The application of computer science to the interpretation and management of biological data.

Biopsy—A small tissue sample.

Borderline leprosy—This form of the disease is characterized by the presence of single or multiple skin lesions with ill-defined or indistinct borders. Many satellite lesions emerge around the larger ones. As suggested by the name, the nerve structure shows an intermediate kind of pathology, with some damage, but not as much as is seen in the tuberculoid form.

Cell mediated immunity—A type of immunity that operates through a type of white blood cell called a T cell. During cell-mediated immune responses, cells that can destroy other cells become active. Their destructive activity is limited to cells that are either infected with, or are producing, a specific antigen.

Cytotoxic—Having a toxic, or deadly, effect on cells.

Endemic—Native to, or restricted to a given place or population.

Gangrenous—Containing dead soft tissue, due to loss of blood supply.

Genomic sequencing—The sequencing of all DNA.

Granulomas—Masses or nodules of chronically inflamed tissue, which are usually associated with an infective process.

Humoral immunity—Type of immunity that principally operates through a type of white blood cell called a B cell, which originates in bone marrow and the spleen. During humoral immune responses, proteins called antibodies, which can stick to and destroy antigens, appear in the blood and other body fluids.

Hyperpigmented—Areas of skin that become darker or redder than the rest of the skin.

Hypopigmented—Areas of skin that get discolored or lose their normal color.

Laminin—A protein specifically found in nerve tissue.

Leonine facies—Lion-like facial features.

Leprologist—A physician experienced in the study and treatment of leprosy.

Lepromatous leprosy—The more easily spread of the two forms of leprosy. This more severe form produces large disfiguring nodules.

Macrophages—Specialized immune cells that can engulf other cells or pathogens.

Major histocompatibility complex (MHC)—A set of cellular surface proteins/antigens that are specific for an organism and play a major role in identifying similar tissue and rejecting tissue from other organisms.

Morbidity—Illness or suffering caused by a disease.

Mortality—Deaths caused by a disease or any other agent.

Multibacillary leprosy—*See* **lepromatous leprosy.**

Neuropathy—A disease or abnormality of the neural system.

Nucleus—The eucaryotic cell organelle that is surrounded by a double membrane and contains all of that cell's genetic material.

Obligate intracellular parasite—A parasite which cannot survive outside a living cell.

Osmotic lysis—Rupturing of a cell when placed in a dilute environment.

Paleobiologists—Scientists who study the biology of fossil organisms.

Paleo-epidemiologists—Scientists who study disease in fossil organisms.

Papule—A small, solid, often inflamed elevation of the skin that does not contain pus.

Glossary

Pasteurization—The process of heating milk and other liquids to destroy microorganisms that can cause spoilage or disease.

Paucibacillary leprosy—Type of leprosy in which the nerve architecture is destroyed and in which there can be formation of granulomas in nerves.

Peptidoglycan—A large polymer composed of long polysaccharide chains that are linked to each other. They provide much of the strength and rigidity of the bacterial cell walls.

Phagocytosis—The engulfing, and usually the destruction of particulate matter by phagocytes.

Polymerase chain reaction (PCR)—An *in vitro* technique used to synthesize large quantities of specific nucleotide sequences from small amounts of DNA.

Prokaryote—Organisms that lack a true membrane bound nucleus.

Pseudogenes—Parts of DNA; similar to genes of other organisms but are not functional.

Ribosome—The organelle where protein synthesis occurs.

Schwann cell—A type of glial cell of the peripheral nervous system that helps separate and insulate nerve cells.

Thymus—A small glandular organ located behind the breastbone.

Transfer RNA (tRNA)—A small RNA that binds an amino acid and delivers it to the ribosome for protein synthesis.

Tuberculoid leprosy—The more benign type of leprosy that affects the nerves; often leads to numbness (usually of the extremities). Affects the peripheral nerves and, sometimes, the surrounding skin on the face, arms, legs, and buttocks.

CHAPTER 1:
HISTORICAL OVERVIEW

1 "Leprosy: History and Incidence," Encyclopedia.com. Available online at http://www.encyclopedia.com/html/section/leprosy_HistoryandIncidence.asp

2 The Leprosy Mission International, Available online at http://www.leprosymission.org

3 Leprosy Sufferers Need Compassion, "Forum on Leprosy." Available online at http://www.webspawner.com/users/LEPROSY/

CHAPTER 3:
LEPROSY AROUND
THE WORLD

4 Sharon Lerner. "Cases of leprosy on the rise in U.S.," *The New York Times*, February 20, 2003, available online at International Herald Tribune, http://www.iht.com/articles/87291.html

5 World Health Organization International. "Elimination of Leprosy as a Public Health Problem." Available online at http://www.who.int/lep/

6 American Leprosy Missions. "Angola: Facts." Available online at http://www.leprosy.org/PROJangola.html

7 Ibid.

8 World Health Organization International. "Global Leprosy Situation." Available online at http://www.cefpas.it/fad/fad/1global.htm

9 Ibid.

10 World Health Organization International. "Weekly epidemiological record." January 4, 2002. Available online at http://www.who.int/docstore/wer/pdf/2002/wer7701.pdf

11 World Health Organization International. "Global Leprosy Situation." Available online at http://www.cefpas.it/fad/fad/1global.htm

CHAPTER 6:
CONTROLLING
THE DISEASE

12 "Leprosy research in the post-genome era". Available online at http://www.lepra.org.uk/review/Mar01/pp8-22.pdf

13 Ibid.

14 American Cancer Society. "Thalidomide Makes News Again: New Research on How Thalidomide May Help the Cancer Patients." October 6, 1998. Available online at http://www.cancer.org/docroot/NWS/content/NWS_1_1x_Thalidomide_Makes_News_Again.asp

CHAPTER 7:
UNDERSTANDING THE
M. LEPRAE BACILLUS

15 San Francisco State University, Department of Geography. "The Biogeography of the Nine-Banded Armadillo," December 7, 1999. Available online at http://bss.sfsu.edu/geog/bholzman/courses/fall99projects/armadillo.htm

16 Cole ST et al. "Massive gene decay in the leprosy bacillus" *Nature* 2001, 409: 1007–1011

CHAPTER 8:
ONGOING REFORMS
AND THE FUTURE

17 "Baba Changing the Lives of Ostracized Lepers." Available online at http://www.brightindia.com/mymite.html

Bibliography

American Cancer Society. "Thalidomide Makes News Again: New Research on How Thalidomide May Help the Cancer Patients." October 6, 1998. Available online at http://www.cancer.org/docroot/NWS/content/NWS _1_1x_Thalidomide_Makes_News_Again.asp

American Leprosy Missions. "Angola: Facts." Available online at http://www .leprosy.org/PROJangola.html

"Baba Changing the Lives of Ostracized Lepers." Available online at http://www.brightindia.com/mymite.html

"Leprosy: History and Incidence." Encyclopia.com. Available online at http://www.encyclopedia.com/html/section/leprosy_HistoryandIncidence .asp

Leprosy Mission International. Available online at http://www.leprosymission .org

"Leprosy research in the post-genome era." Available online at http://www .lepra.org.uk/review/Mar01/pp8-22.pdf

Leprosy Sufferers Need Compassion. "Forum on Leprosy." Available online at http://www.webspawner.com/users/LEPROSY/

Lerner, Sharon. "Cases of leprosy on the rise in U.S." *The New York Times*, February 20, 2003, available online at International Herald Tribune, http://www.iht.com/articles/87291.html

San Francisco State University. Department of Geography. "The Biogeography of the Nine-Banded Armadillo." December 7, 1999. Available online at http://bss.sfsu.edu/geog/bholzman/courses/fall99 projects/armadillo.htm

World Health Organization International. "Elimination of Leprosy as a Public Health Problem." Available online at http://www.who.int/lep/

———. "Global Leprosy Situation." Available online at http://www.cefpas.it/ fad/fad/1global.htm

———. "Weekly epidemiological record." January 4, 2002. Available online at http://www.who.int/docstore/wer/pdf/2002/wer7701.pdf

Further Reading

ADe Mallac, M.J. *Hansen's Disease: The Shared Paradigm*. East Sussex, England: Book Guild, Ltd, 2001.

Donnelly, Karen. *Leprosy*. New York: Rosen Publishing Group, 2001.

Farrow, John. *Damien the Leper*. Image, 1998.

Gaudet, Marcia. *Carville: Remembering Leprosy in America*. Jackson, MS: University Press of Mississippi, 2004.

Job, C.K. *Leprosy: Diagnosis and Management*. New Dehli, India: Indian Leprosy Association, 1975.

Kappor, P. *Guide to Leprosy and Leprosy Control*. India: J.M. Mehta, 1977.

Stewart, Richard. *Leper Priest of Moloka'i: The Father Damien Story*. Honolulu: HI: University of Hawaii Press, 2000.

Websites

American Leprosy Missions
http://www.leprosy.org/

World Health Organization—Leprosy Information
http://www.who.int/lep/

Centers for Disease Control—Hansen's Disease (Leprosy)
http://www.cdc.gov/ncidod/dbmd/diseaseinfo/hansens_t.htm

Index

Picture Credits

About the Author

Alfica Sehgal, Ph.D., is currently completing her postdoctoral research at Johns Hopkins Medical School in Baltimore Maryland. She received her Ph.D. in molecular parasitology from Tata Institute of Fundamental Research in Mumbai, India. She received her first postdoctoral research training at Yale University School of Medicine in New Haven, Connecticut. During her Ph.D. and post-doctoral training, she performed extensive molecular level research on parasites like Plasmodium and Toxoplasma. Sehgal is interested in studying the basic biological mechanisms in different organisms and applying that knowledge to improve pharmacological and diagnostic methods.

About the Founding Editor

The late I. Edward Alcamo was a Distinguished Teaching Professor of Microbiology at the State University of New York at Farmingdale. Alcamo studied biology at Iona College in New York and earned his M.S. and Ph.D. degrees in microbiology at St. John's University, also in New York. He had taught at Farmingdale for over 30 years. In 2000, Alcamo won the Carski Award for Distinguished Teaching in Microbiology, the highest honor for microbiology teachers in the United States. He was a member of the American Society for Microbiology, the National Association of Biology Teachers, and the American Medical Writers Association. Alcamo authored numerous books on the subjects of microbiology, AIDS, and DNA technology as well as the award-winning textbook *Fundamentals of Microbiology*, now in its sixth edition.

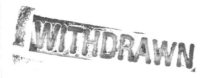